GLUTEN-FREE
food for kids

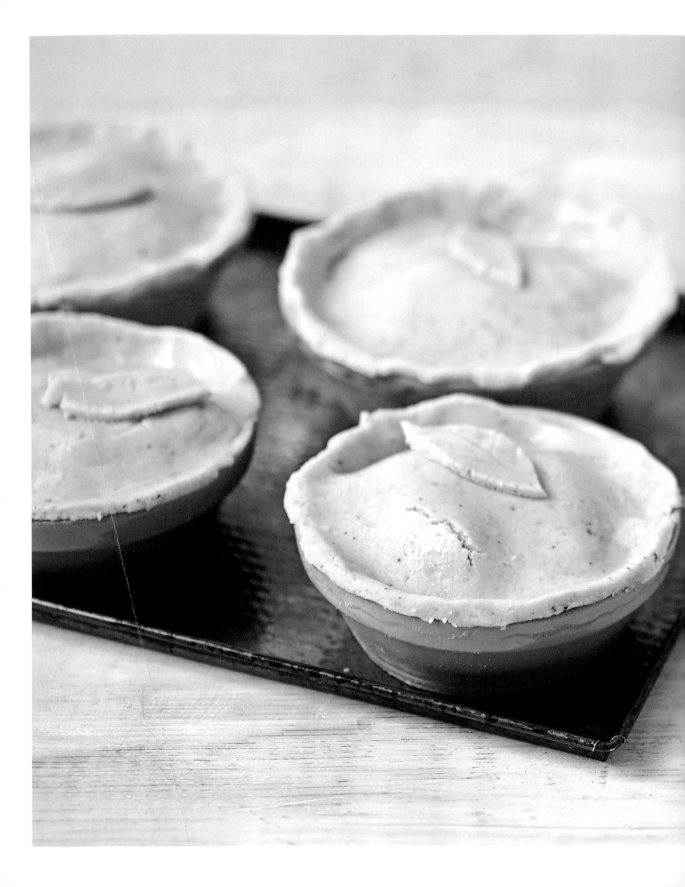

GLUTEN-FREE
food for kids

More than 100 quick & easy recipes for coeliac children

Louise Blair

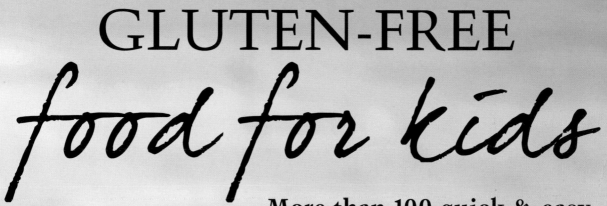

hamlyn

An Hachette UK Company
www.hachette.co.uk

First published in Great Britain in 2015 by
Hamlyn, a division of Octopus Publishing Group Ltd
Carmelite House
50 Victoria Embankment
London EC4Y 0DZ
www.octopusbooks.co.uk

Louise Blair asserts the moral right to be identified as the author of this work

ISBN 978 0 60063 107 1

A CIP catalogue record for this book is available from the British Library

Printed and bound in China

10 9 8 7 6 5 4 3 2 1

Both metric and imperial measurements have been given in all recipes. Use one set of measurements only, and not a mixture of both.

Standard level spoon measurements are used in all recipes.
1 tablespoon = one 15 ml spoon
1 teaspoon = one 5 ml spoon

Ovens should be preheated to the specified temperature – if using a fan-assisted oven, follow the manufacturer's instructions for adjusting the time and temperature.

Fresh herbs should be used unless otherwise stated.

Medium eggs should be used unless otherwise stated.

The Department of Health advises that eggs should not be consumed raw. This book contains some dishes made with raw or lightly cooked eggs. It is prudent for vulnerable people such as pregnant and nursing mothers, invalids, the elderly, babies and young children to avoid uncooked or lightly cooked dishes made with eggs. Once prepared, these dishes should be kept refrigerated and used promptly.

This book includes dishes made with nuts and nut derivatives. It is advisable for those with known allergic reactions to nuts and nut derivatives and those who may be potentially vulnerable to these allergies to avoid dishes made with nuts and nut oils. It is also prudent to check the labels of pre-prepared ingredients for the possible inclusion of nut derivatives.

contents

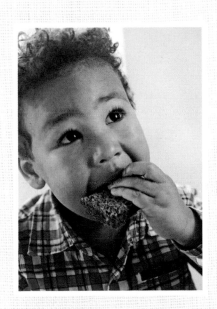
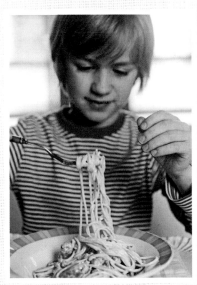
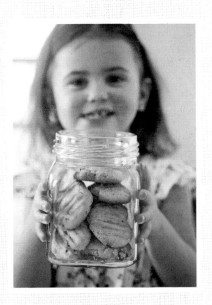

introduction

Being diagnosed with a lifelong condition such as coeliac disease can be extremely daunting to an adult and for a child it can be even more stressful and upsetting. This book aims to show you and your child that such a diagnosis needn't be the end of the world, and your child need not feel different or excluded from the things that others take for granted.

If you have a child who has been diagnosed with coeliac disease, remember that there is a lot of assistance out there to help. Once your child has received the correct support and education and follows a gluten-free diet, symptoms will improve and he or she can live a very normal life.

What is gluten?

Gluten is a protein that is found in a number of grains including wheat, barley and rye. Due to cross-contamination during the processing of some oats, they too can contain gluten. Gluten gives dough its 'stretch', helping give stability and shape and giving the end product its desirable 'chewiness'. Given that grains containing gluten are the main ingredient in many popular and staple food items such as breads, biscuits and cakes, being told that these are now a 'no-go' area may seem overwhelming or impossible and finding suitable alternatives challenging. What we aim to show you in this book is that there is life beyond gluten! And a delicious one, too.

What is coeliac disease?

Contrary to common misconceptions, coeliac disease is not a food allergy or a food intolerance, it is an autoimmune disease whereby the body makes antibodies against the protein 'gluten'. Antibodies that are usually responsible for attacking bacteria and viruses detect the gluten and attack it, thus causing inflammation of the lining of the small intestine.

Causes and symptoms

The lining of the small intestine is covered with millions of finger-like projections called villi. When antibodies attack the gluten in foods they cause inflammation, which in turn flattens the villi, meaning that nutrients from food cannot be so readily absorbed. This can result in deficiencies including anaemia.

Other symptoms range from mild to severe and can include diarrhoea, bloating, abdominal pain, excess wind, and tiredness or weakness. Often the symptoms of coeliac disease are confused with irritable bowel syndrome (IBS) or a wheat intolerance, as they manifest themselves similarly. Symptoms can also vary from person to person: in infants, coeliac disease presents as a failure to thrive; in children, it can cause a lack of appetite, altered bowel habits and anaemia; and within the adult population symptoms

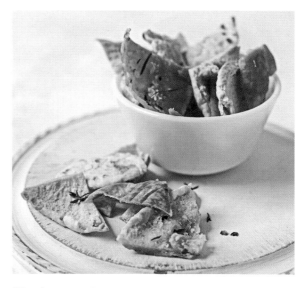

pitta crisps, page 47

include anaemia, diarrhoea, chronic tiredness and lethargy, weight loss and other abdominal abnormalities. Other body systems can also be affected manifesting as headaches, hair loss, tooth enamel erosion and joint pain. Long-term problems caused by untreated or undiagnosed coeliac disease can result in the following:

- Infertility in women, including recurrent miscarriage
- Poor growth of babies during pregnancy
- Osteoporosis – thinning of bones
- An increased risk of bowel cancer, intestinal lymphoma and cancer of the oesophagus.

A gluten-free diet reduces these complications as well as other associated conditions such as mouth ulcers and dermatitis herpetiformis. Sticking to a gluten-free diet will also reduce the risk of any cancers associated with coeliac disease and bring these occurances in line with statistics for the normal population.

Who suffers from coeliac disease?

Almost 1 in 100 people in the UK are affected by coeliac disease, but it is thought that at least 60 per cent remain undiagnosed. Anyone, at any age, can develop coeliac disease and it is most commonly diagnosed in people aged between 40 and 50. About 1 in 4 cases are first diagnosed in people aged over 60. Coeliac disease can be hereditary – if you have a close family member who has coeliac disease, then you have a 1 in 10 chance of having or developing coeliac disease. If your child has another autoimmune disease – for example, some thyroid diseases, rheumatoid arthritis and Type 1 diabetes – then he or she is also more predisposed to having or developing coeliac disease.

Diagnosis and treatment

If you suspect your child has coeliac disease, don't remove gluten from his or her diet immediately. First of all, consult your doctor, who will carry out a simple blood test to detect if the antibody against gluten is present. If this blood test is positive, your child may be referred for a biopsy of the lining of the small intestine to see if the tell-tale signs of coeliac disease are present. Cutting out gluten before your child is tested may give a negative result.

If your child tests positive then the next step is to completely cut out gluten from his or her diet for life. Symptoms will usually disappear within a couple of weeks and the small intestine will begin to repair itself. Symptoms will return, however, even if only a tiny amount of gluten is consumed. Your doctor should refer you to a dietitian who can give you advice on how to deal with coeliac disease and what your child should and shouldn't eat. Coeliac UK (www.coeliac.org.uk) is another important port of call – it provides not only advice but also a Food and Drink Directory that lists all gluten-free foods. Manufacturers occasionally change ingredients or suppliers and therefore a product that was previously gluten-free may change to contain gluten. Coeliac UK updates its lists monthly so that you are able to keep up to date with any changes.

In the UK, gluten-free food is available on prescription for people with coeliac disease. These foods are generally staples in the diet, such as bread and pasta, rather than biscuits and cake items. Remember that left untreated, coeliac disease can cause anaemia and osteoporosis, so don't just ignore it.

Children and coeliac disease

Children and their siblings of all ages need to recognize their diagnosis, understanding why their bodies act in a different way when exposed to gluten and how this relates to how well they feel. Children have an amazing ability to adapt and with the right help and support this lifestyle change should be easily attained. Coeliac UK (see above) is an excellent resource and is on hand to provide guidance and advice.

A meeting with school teachers, catering staff and the school nurse is essential. Coeliac UK can provide a 'School Pack' that covers all aspects of your child's school life and how the school can help. Schools are required to make arrangements to support children so meeting all involved is a good way to ensure that this is done and that appropriate support is in place.

The most important thing to remember is that your child is not alone – there are lots of other kids in the same situation and many people to help and guide them.

Introducing a gluten-free diet

Bearing in mind that gluten is present in all wheat, barley and rye products, and very often in oats through cross-contamination, careful thought needs to be given to shopping for, preparing and cooking a gluten-free diet for your child.

Most manufacturers label products that are gluten-free and may use the Crossed Grain symbol, or their version of this symbol. Even if the packaging doesn't show you the information in this way, looking at the list of ingredients will identify if any products containing gluten are used.

Some foods that contain gluten are obvious – breads, cakes, pastries, biscuits and pasta, for instance. Others, such as processed foods including some sweets, chocolate, soups, crisps and sausages, may also contain gluten, so a good study of food labels is essential. But don't panic! Take a look round at all the wonderful foods that are naturally gluten-free (see right) and you will see that these can be used to make delicious meals. A quick read through the recipes in this book will also reveal that gluten-free cooking can still be exciting, simple, easy and delicious.

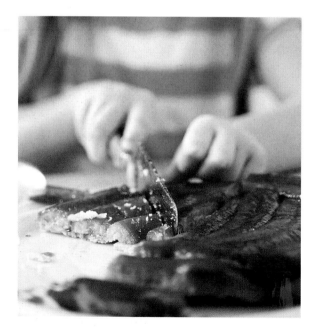

banana tarte tartin, page 122

Naturally gluten-free foods
- Fruits and vegetables, including potatoes
- Unprocessed meat, poultry and fish (including shellfish)
- Unprocessed cheeses, butter, milk and plain milk products including cream
- Eggs
- Tofu
- Cooking oils
- Sugar, bicarbonate of soda, cream of tartar and yeast
- Plain nuts, seeds and pulses
- Rice and associated rice products, such as rice noodles and rice flour
- Gluten-free grains and their associated products, such as buckwheat noodles, polenta, cornflour and cornmeal*
- Natural yogurt
- Vinegars
- Fats
- Coffee and tea
- Herbs and spices

*NB: Some naturally gluten-free grains are milled with wheat, barley and rye, and therefore may be cross-contaminated with grains that do contain gluten; always read the packet label.

Foods that contain gluten
- Wheat, barley and rye and their products, such as pasta, wheat noodles, bulgar wheat and couscous
- Breads, cakes, biscuits, breakfast cereals and snacks/confectionery containing wheat, barley and rye flour
- Baking powder
- Foods covered in batter, breadcrumbs or dusted with flour
- Barley water/squash and malted milk drinks
- Some mustard products may contain wheat as a thickener
- Chinese soy sauce, which is traditionally made from fermented wheat
- Stuffing mixes
- Some ready-made seasonings, sauces, soups, gravy granules and stock cubes
- Some sausages contain wheat husk

Gluten-free shop-bought alternatives

As well as the basic foodstuffs that are gluten-free, you can also buy pre-prepared food items that use gluten-free ingredients as a substitute for those containing gluten. As consumers have become increasingly aware of the benefits of a gluten-free diet, food manufacturers have been creating a growing range of gluten-free products, such as breads, biscuits and pasta. Many of these products have come a long way from the bland, poor-quality gluten-free foods of years gone by and are often available even at smaller stores.

Gluten-free products are not always quite the same as traditional goods, however, as it is gluten that gives bread its elasticity and cakes their spring. If you try one product and your child doesn't like it, don't despair – try another brand or get baking yourself! You will be surprised when you sample some of the carefully selected recipes in this book that gluten-free ingredients can replicate fairly closely many of the foods that contain gluten.

Store-cupboard essentials

As mentioned before, there are many naturally gluten-free products such as unprocessed meat and fish, dairy foods, fresh fruit and vegetables, rice and pulses. However, you will need to prepare other common foods that are not normally gluten-free – such as white sauce, gravy, cakes, breads and pasta and noodle dishes – using gluten-free ingredients. If you look out for and stock up on some of the following items you will be able to make all the recipes in this book whenever you wish.

Flours

As well as certain flour mixes, there are other gluten-free flours that can be used for baking and cooking, such as rice, chickpea, potato, soya, corn, buckwheat and millet. If these flours are not available in your local supermarket, they can usually be found in health-food stores or can be ordered online. You don't need to buy them all, however – for general all-purpose use, I find rice flour a great all-rounder and cornflour is good for sauces and thickening in stews, although it is worth experimenting with other flours as well. This book primarily uses rice flour and cornflour.

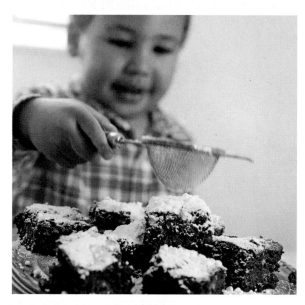

banana & peanut brownies, page 96

Xanthan gum

A powder that greatly aids gluten-free baking, xanthan gum, to some extent, replaces the elastic qualities that gluten-free flours lack. Adding a little to gluten-free flours makes bread less crumbly and gluten-free pastry easier to roll and handle. It's available in specialist health-food stores and in some supermarkets. I have only used xanthan gum in these recipes where it is really needed, opting to use a variety or mix of other flours to get the best results. It is often used in bread recipes and scones, as well as cakes and biscuits.

Gluten-free baking powder

Standard, shop-bought baking powder contains gluten, but gluten-free baking powder is now widely available in the baking sections of most larger supermarkets. If you prefer, you can make your own gluten-free baking powder with bicarbonate of soda and cream of tartar which are both naturally gluten-free. Simply mix 2 parts bicarbonate of soda with 1 part cream of tartar and use this spoon for spoon in baking, as you would with a standard, shop-bought baking powder.

Pasta and noodles

Gluten-free pastas are becoming more common, and are marketed as such. Rice noodles are gluten-free, as are the varieties of soba noodles that are made entirely from buckwheat.

Grains

Quinoa is a brilliant addition to the diet, providing an excellent source of protein as well as being gluten-free. It is a great substitute for couscous or bulgar wheat in salads and side dishes. Polenta is good for baking and for use as an alternative coating to breadcrumbs. As a form of carbohydrate, it can also be used in place of pasta.

Pulses

Lentils and beans can be used in stews and casseroles, but are also great in salads or as side dishes.

Cheese and dairy

Unprocessed cheeses are gluten-free and brilliant to have on hand in the refrigerator; don't overuse, though, as they are high in fat! Milk and natural, unflavoured yogurts are gluten-free, and it is worth looking at the labels of other dairy products to find gluten-free options.

As with all types of cooking, gluten-free cooking can be a case of trial and error because gluten-free products have different baking qualities and properties. Don't give up if you find that you don't instantly get good results – you will achieve acceptable results eventually. As well as providing a satisfying gluten-free diet for your child, rest assured that the rest of the family will also be more than happy with the recipes in this book.

Cross-contamination

So you have cut out gluten from your child's diet, found your way round the gluten-free products available and have the gluten-free foods list to hand (*see* page 8) ... all should be plain sailing from here. You, your child and your family must be aware, however, that cross-contamination is easy: by spreading butter that has been contaminated with 'normal' breadcrumbs on gluten-free toast; by using

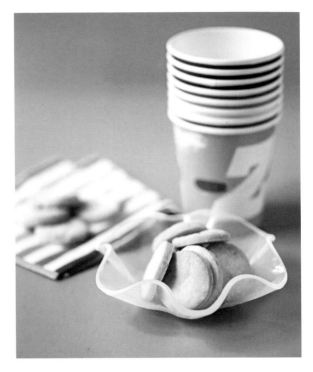

cheesy bites, page 126

the same toaster for gluten-free and 'normal' bread; or by stirring a gluten-free dish with a spoon that has been stirring gravy made with wheat flour. Even small amounts of gluten can cause the symptoms of coeliac disease to return. Make the following simple but important tips a part of your cooking routine in order to prevent cross-contamination:

- Store gluten-free flours separately
- Use separate utensils to prepare gluten-free food
- Keep a 'gluten-free' sieve, rolling pin, pastry brush and chopping board
- Wash everything well and clean surfaces before cooking and eating

It is often easier to cook one gluten-free dish for the whole family – it takes less time and involves less risk of cross-contamination.

Day-to-day life

Avoiding gluten is for life. If your child eats gluten again, symptoms will return. Even small amounts of gluten can re-sensitize the gut. To avoid symptoms returning and further complications, your child must be strict about avoiding all foods that contain gluten (*see* page 8).

Start the way you mean to go on. Involve your child in choosing suitable foodstuffs and ingredients and how to prepare them without risking cross-contamination. Mark foods with stickers as to whether gluten-free or not and make sure they understand, if they are old enough, about cross-contamination (see left). If involved from the beginning it will quickly become routine and your child will be more aware when away from you.

Holding children's parties

Keep it simple and serve the same food for all the children. There is a great selection of party foods in this cookbook, including sausage rolls, cakes, cheesy bites and biscuits. If you don't have time to prepare it all yourself, however, you can supplement it with gluten-free shop-bought foods, such as vegetables to make crudités to serve with gluten-free dips, gluten-free sausages and fresh fruit. There are several cake recipes in this book, such as the Chocolate Sponge with Buttercream on page 134, which can be easily adapted to your child's requests.

Fizzy drinks, fruit juices and most fruit cordials do not contain gluten, but check any cloudy drinks as these may contain barley.

Away from home

Parties and play dates

When your child is going on a play date or to a party, you will need to liaise with the other parents or organizer. While it is important to give your child the independence to manage his or her own diet, when away from home your child may not be too sure about all the food on offer. For peace of mind, you may find it easier to pack up some food for your child. Ask what types of party food are being prepared so you can substitute similar gluten-free versions. Perhaps you could bring along gluten-free alternatives for everyone to try so your child feels included.

Eating out

Check the menu of restaurants where you plan to eat and make sure that staff are aware of your child's condition prior to your visit. Hidden gluten can be in sauces, coatings (for example, breadcrumbs), gravy and stock cubes. Many chefs are happy to cook something off the menu for your child with your advice.

Cooking at school

With careful planning there is no reason why your child cannot take part in cooking at school. Get a step ahead of the game and liaise with the class teacher to ensure that you child is able to use utensils that haven't come into contact with gluten. You could also provide a gluten-free recipe for the whole class to make, which will help to eliminate the risk of cross-contamination.

Making mistakes

If your child eats gluten by mistake, some symptoms will usually start to appear a few hours after eating and the effects can last from a few hours to several days depending on your child's sensitivity to what he or she has eaten. You may want to treat the symptoms or prefer to wait until they naturally get better. If your child is experiencing diarrhoea or is vomiting, it is important to keep him or her well hydrated by making sure they drink lots of water. Some people also find that taking medication to treat constipation, diarrhoea or headaches can ease symptoms, so speak to your pharmacist or GP. The most important thing is to get your child back on to a gluten-free diet as soon as possible to try to prevent further symptoms. If your child's symptoms are very severe or do not improve, you should discuss this with your GP.

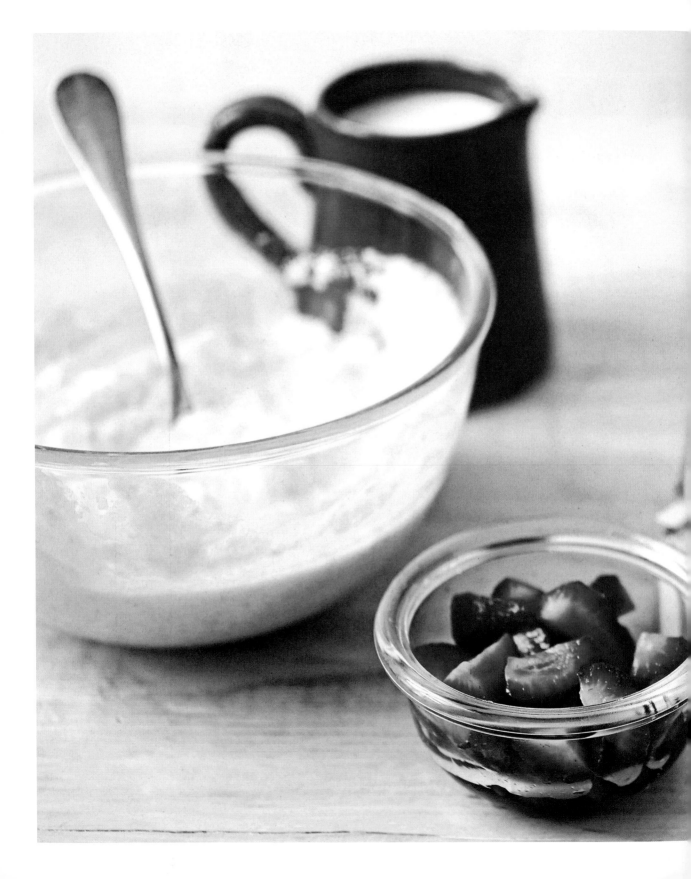

breakfast

yogurt & berry smoothie

Serves 4

Preparation time 5 minutes

300 ml (½ pint) natural yogurt

500 g (1 lb) fresh or frozen mixed summer berries, defrosted if frozen, plus extra to decorate

4 tablespoons millet flakes

3 tablespoons clear honey

300 ml (½ pint) cranberry juice

Millet flakes are an excellent source of magnesium, while the berries provide plenty of Vitamin C for healthy kids.

1 Place all the ingredients in a food processor or a blender and blitz until smooth.

2 Pour into 4 glasses, decorate with a few extra whole berries and serve immediately.

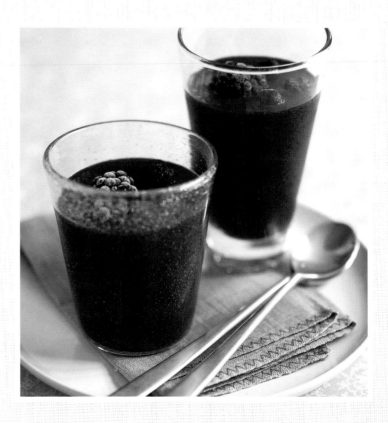

tropical fruit smoothie

Serves 4

Preparation time 10 minutes

1 mango, peeled, stoned and chopped

2 kiwifruits, peeled and chopped

1 banana, cut into chunks

425 g (14 oz) can pineapple chunks or pieces in natural juice

450 ml (¾ pint) orange or apple juice

handful of ice cubes

This is like sunshine in a glass and provides an easy breakfast on the go, or mid-morning energy boost.

1 Place all the ingredients in a food processor or blender and blitz until smooth.

2 Pour into 4 glasses and serve immediately.

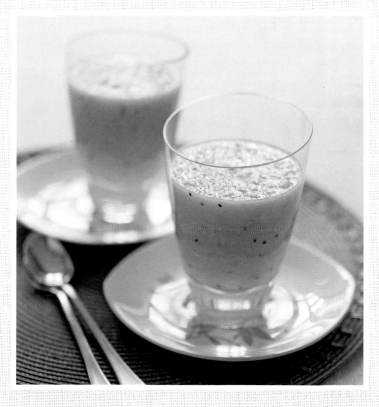

bircher muesli

Serves 4

**Preparation time 5 minutes, plus
  overnight soaking**

200 g (7 oz) buckwheat flakes

300 ml (½ pint) milk

100 ml (3½ fl oz) apple juice

1 apple, peeled and grated

2 tablespoons clear honey

100 g (3½ oz) ready-to-eat dried fruit, such
  as mango, apricots or sultanas

100 g (3½ oz) hazelnuts, toasted and
  roughly chopped

poached or canned fruit, such as peaches
  or berries, to serve

1 Mix together the buckwheat flakes, milk, apple juice and grated apple in a bowl. Cover and leave to soak overnight.

2 To serve, stir the honey, dried fruit and nuts into the muesli mixture. Spoon into bowls, then top with the poached or canned fruit and serve.

Tips and tricks
You can try this recipe with any of your favourite dried fruit and nuts, or add a bit of dried coconut for a tropical flavour.

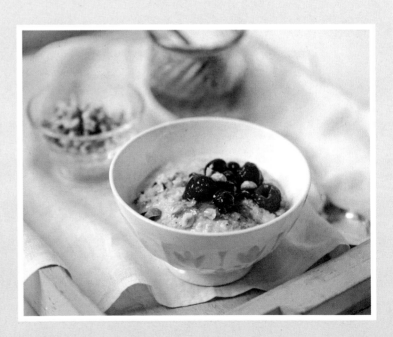

buckwheat porridge

Serves 4

Preparation time 5 minutes

Cooking time 5 minutes

200 g (7 oz) buckwheat flakes

1 ripe banana, chopped

½ teaspoon ground cinnamon

100 g (3½ oz) sultanas

200 ml (7 fl oz) milk

200 ml (7 fl oz) water

clear honey, to serve

200 g (7 oz) mixed berries, to serve

To vary the porridge, try replacing the banana with a chopped pear and serve with chopped toasted walnuts and honey.

1 Place all the ingredients in a saucepan over a low heat and bring to a simmer, then cook gently for 3–4 minutes until the flakes are tender.

2 Blend briefly with a stick blender, then serve drizzled with a little honey.

breakfast cereal bars

Makes 16

Preparation time 10 minutes

Cooking time 35 minutes

100 g (3½ oz) butter, softened, plus extra
  for greasing

25 g (1 oz) soft light brown sugar

2 tablespoons golden syrup

125 g (4 oz) millet flakes

50 g (2 oz) quinoa

50 g (2 oz) dried cherries or cranberries

75 g (3 oz) sultanas

25 g (1 oz) sunflower seeds

25 g (1 oz) sesame seeds

25 g (1 oz) linseeds

40 g (1½ oz) unsweetened desiccated
  coconut

2 eggs, lightly beaten

1 Grease a 28 x 20 cm (11 x 8 inch) shallow baking tin.

2 Beat together the butter, sugar and syrup in a large bowl until creamy. Add all the remaining ingredients and beat well until combined.

3 Spoon the mixture into the prepared tin and level the surface with the back of the spoon. Place in a preheated oven, 180°C (350°F), Gas Mark 4, for 35 minutes until deep golden. Leave to cool in the tin.

4 Turn out on to a wooden board and carefully cut into 16 fingers using a serrated knife. Store in an airtight container for up to 5 days.

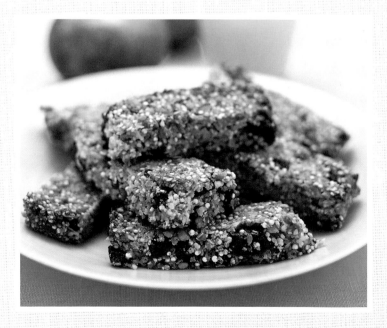

chewy tropical squares

Makes 9

Preparation time 10 minutes

Cooking time 20 minutes

butter, for greasing

100 g (3½ oz) dates, chopped

50 g (2 oz) dried mango, chopped

100 g (3½ oz) ready-to-eat dried apricots, chopped

100 ml (3½ fl oz) orange juice

50 g (2 oz) almonds, skin on

175 g (6 oz) ground almonds

100 g (3½ oz) mixed sunflower and pumpkin seeds

2 tablespoons desiccated coconut

2 tablespoons maple syrup

1 Lightly grease a 20 cm (8 inch) square baking tin.

2 Place the fruits and orange juice in a bowl. Soak for 5 minutes.

3 Transfer the mixture to a food processor or blender, add the whole almonds and blend briefly so the mixture retains some texture. Stir in all the remaining ingredients, except the syrup.

4 Press the mixture into the prepared tin and place in a preheated oven, 180°C (350°F), Gas Mark 4, for 20 minutes until golden.

5 Brush over the maple syrup, then mark into 9 squares and leave to cool in the tin before turning out and breaking into the squares.

6 Store in an airtight container for 2–3 days.

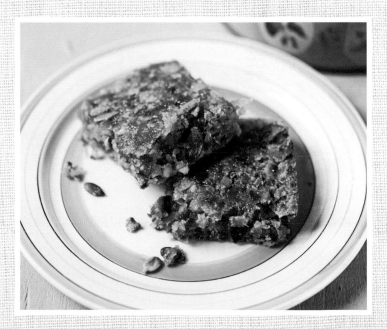

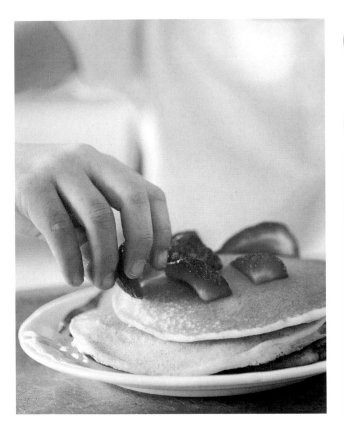
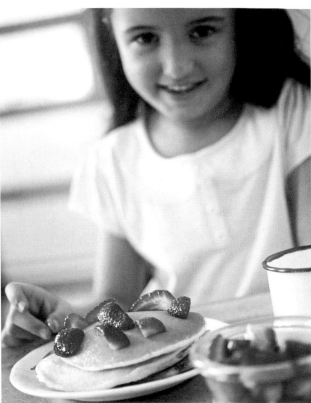
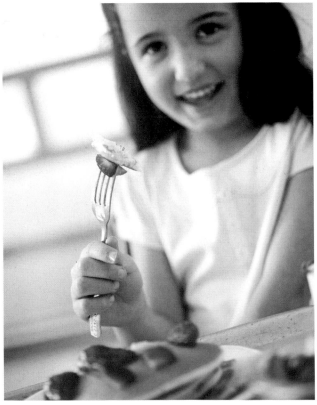
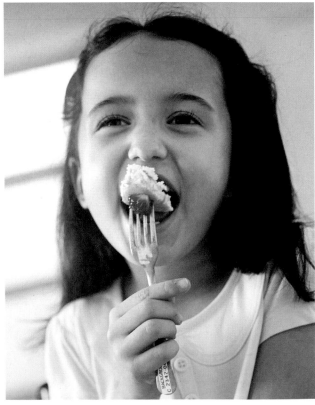

dreamy new york pancakes

Makes 8

Preparation time 10 minutes

Cooking time 10–15 minutes

3 large eggs, separated

125 g (4 oz) brown rice flour

1 teaspoon gluten-free baking powder

1 tablespoon caster sugar

150 ml (¼ pint) milk

butter, for frying

Topping

450 g (14½ oz) strawberries, hulled and halved

1 tablespoon caster sugar

You can use any fruit, such as blackberries, plums, cherries or fresh apricots, to top the pancakes. If you prefer savoury pancakes for breakfast, try serving these with crisp streaky bacon rashers drizzled with maple syrup.

1 Whisk together the egg yolks, flour, baking powder, sugar and milk in a large bowl. Whisk the egg whites until stiff in a separate clean bowl, then fold into the flour mixture.

2 Stir together the strawberries and sugar and set aside while cooking the pancakes.

3 Heat a little butter in a frying pan, spoon in tablespoons of the pancake batter and cook for 1–2 minutes on each side until golden and puffed up. Remove from the pan and keep warm while you cook the remaining pancakes.

4 Serve the pancakes topped with the strawberries.

Tips and tricks

It is important to use the batter immediately as it will become too runny if left.

sweet eggy bread with cinnamon apples

Serves 4

Preparation time 5 minutes

Cooking time 5 minutes

2 eggs

1 tablespoon caster sugar

2 tablespoons milk

few drops of vanilla extract

4 thick slices of gluten-free bread

25 g (1 oz) butter

Cinnamon apples

knob of butter, for frying

2 dessert apples, peeled, cored and finely sliced

1 tablespoon caster sugar

squeeze of lemon juice

½ tablespoon ground cinnamon

This is also delicious served as a dessert with dollops of vanilla ice cream, cream or crème fraîche.

1 Beat together the eggs, sugar, milk and vanilla extract in a shallow bowl. Dip the slices of bread into the egg mixture, ensuring they are fully coated in the mixture.

2 Heat the butter in a large nonstick frying pan, add the eggy bread and fry for 1–2 minutes on each side until golden. Remove from the pan and keep warm.

3 Meanwhile, place all the cinnamon apple ingredients in a saucepan and cook gently for 4–5 minutes until the apples are just tender.

4 Serve the eggy bread topped with the cinnamon apples.

savoury eggy bread

Serves 4

Preparation time 5 minutes

Cooking time 5 minutes

2 eggs, beaten

2 tablespoons milk

2 tablespoons grated Parmesan cheese

2 tablespoons snipped chives

4 thick slices of gluten-free bread

25 g (1 oz) butter

salt and black pepper

Try making this with the Basic White Loaf (*see* page 110) – it works well in this recipe. The eggy bread is delicious served topped with a poached egg, some crisp bacon or cooked gluten-free sausage.

1 Beat together the eggs, milk, Parmesan and chives in a shallow bowl and season well. Dip the slices of bread into the egg mixture, ensuring they are fully coated in the mixture.

2 Heat the butter in a large nonstick frying pan, add the eggy bread and fry for 1–2 minutes on each side until golden.

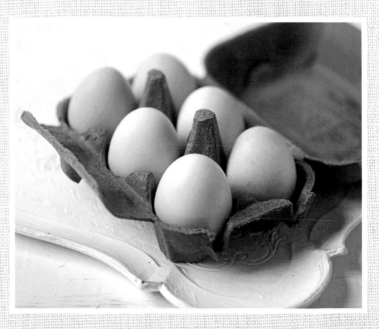

banana & date bread

Makes 1 loaf

Preparation time 10 minutes

Cooking time 1 hour

100 g (3½ oz) butter, softened, plus extra
  for greasing

125 g (4 oz) dates, chopped

½ teaspoon bicarbonate of soda

100 ml (3½ fl oz) boiling water

2 teaspoons gluten-free baking powder

125 g (4 oz) rice flour

50 g (2 oz) cornflour

75 g (3 oz) caster sugar

2 eggs, beaten

4 small ripe bananas, mashed

1 Grease and line a 900 g (2 lb) loaf tin.

2 Place the dates and bicarbonate of soda in a small bowl and pour over the measurement water. Set aside.

3 Beat together all the remaining ingredients in a large bowl. Pour the date mixture into the cake mixture and stir well, then pour into the prepared tin.

4 Place in a preheated oven, 160°C (325°F), Gas Mark 3, for about 1 hour until golden, risen and a skewer inserted into the centre comes out clean. Cool on a wire rack (also delicious served warm).

Tips and tricks

Try adding chocolate chips and a tablespoon of cocoa to the cake mixture for a special treat, or experiment with raisins and other dried fruit if you prefer.

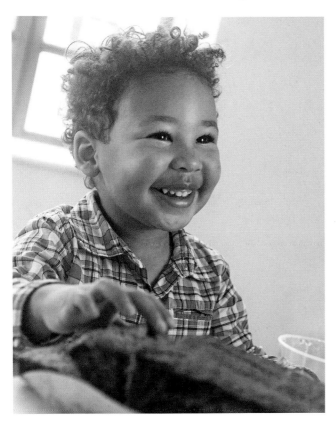
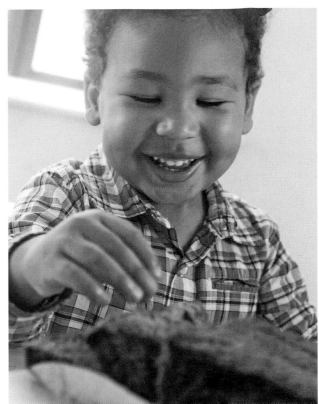
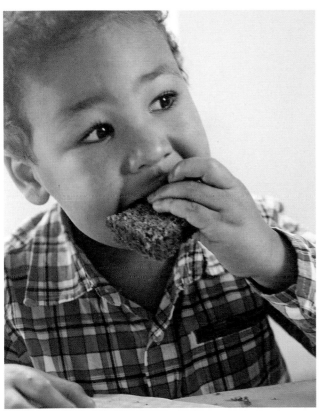
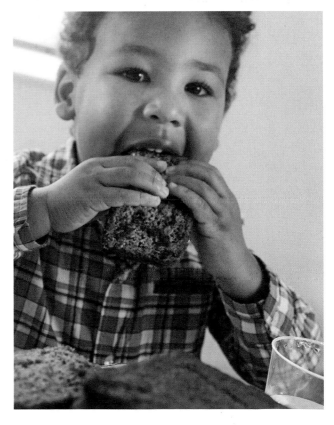

waffles & fresh fruit

Serves 4

Preparation time 5 minutes, plus resting

Cooking time 10 minutes

125 g (4 oz) brown rice flour

125 g (4 oz) gram flour

2 teaspoons gluten-free baking powder

2 tablespoons caster sugar

1½ teaspoons xanthan gum

3 large eggs, beaten

150 ml (¼ pint) double cream

350 ml (12 fl oz) milk

few drops of vanilla extract

150 g (5 oz) butter, melted and cooled

fresh strawberries or blueberries, to serve

If you don't have a waffle iron, then you can make these as pancakes instead.

1 Mix together the flours, baking powder, sugar and xantham gum in a large bowl. Whisk together all the remaining ingredients in a jug, then pour into the dry ingredients and whisk to form a smooth batter. Cover with clingfilm and leave to rest in the refrigerator for at least 1 hour or overnight.

2 Heat a waffle iron until hot, then pour in a small ladle of the batter, ensuring you don't over-fill the iron. Cook according to the manufacturer's instructions until golden. Serve immediately, topped with fresh strawberries or blueberries.

3 Repeat with the remaining batter until all the mixture is used up.

mini tomato & feta omelettes

Makes 12
Preparation time 10 minutes
Cooking time 10 minutes

melted butter, for greasing
4 eggs, beaten
2 tablespoons chopped chives
3 sun-dried tomatoes, finely sliced
75 g (3 oz) feta cheese, crumbled
salt and black pepper

1 Lightly brush a 12-hole mini muffin tray with melted butter.

2 Mix together all the remaining ingredients in a large bowl until just combined.

3 Pour the mixture into the prepared tin and place in a preheated oven, 220°C (425°F), Gas Mark 7, for about 10 minutes until golden and puffed up. Serve warm.

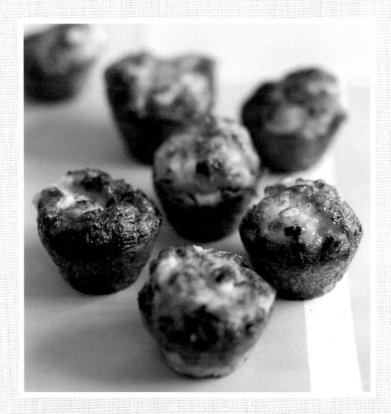

granola & blueberry compote yogurt

Serves 4

Preparation time 10 minutes, plus cooling

Cooking time 20 minutes

300 g (10 oz) blueberries

4 tablespoons apple juice

400 g (13 oz) natural or Greek yogurt

Granola

4 tablespoons maple syrup, plus extra
  to serve

2 tablespoons demerara sugar

2 tablespoons vegetable oil

200 g (7 oz) mixed nuts, such as pecan
  nuts, hazelnuts and almonds, roughly
  chopped

2 tablespoons sunflower seeds

200 g (7 oz) buckwheat flakes

100 g (3½ oz) millet flakes

150 g (5 oz) raisins or other dried fruit

1 Make the granola. Mix together the syrup, sugar and oil in a large bowl, then add the nuts, seeds and flakes and toss until well coated. Tip on to a large baking sheet and place in a preheated oven, 180°C (350°F), Gas Mark 4, for 10 minutes. Stir through the dried fruit and bake for a further 10 minutes.

2 Meanwhile, place the blueberries and apple juice in a small saucepan and cook for a few minutes until the juices begin to run. Leave to cool.

3 Remove the granola from the oven and leave to cool. (It can be stored in an airtight container for up to 1 week.)

4 To serve spoon a little of the yogurt into 4 tall glasses then layer up with the compote and tablespoons of granola. Finishing with a layer of granola.

english breakfast muffins

Makes 12

Preparation time 10 minutes

Cooking time 20–25 minutes

4 streaky bacon rashers

1 gluten-free sausage

2 teaspoons olive oil, for frying

100 g (3½ oz) mushrooms, chopped

250 g (8 oz) brown rice flour

1 teaspoon bicarbonate of soda

2 teaspoons gluten-free baking powder

75 g (3 oz) butter, melted

2 eggs, beaten

150 ml (¼ pint) buttermilk

salt and black pepper

1 Line a 12-hole muffin tray with muffin cases.

2 Cook the bacon and sausage under a preheated grill until cooked through and the bacon is crisp. Leave to cool slightly, then crumble the bacon and thinly slice the sausage.

3 Meanwhile, heat a little oil in a frying pan, add the mushrooms and fry for about 5 minutes until softened.

4 Sift the flour, bicarbonate of soda and baking powder into a large bowl, then add the bacon, sausage and mushrooms and stir together. Whisk together the butter, eggs and buttermilk in a jug and season well, then pour into the dry ingredients and stir until just combined (leave the mixture a little lumpy as this will give a better end result).

5 Spoon the mixture into the muffin cases and place in a preheated oven, 180°C (350°F), Gas Mark 4, for 15–18 minutes until golden and just firm to the touch. Serve warm.

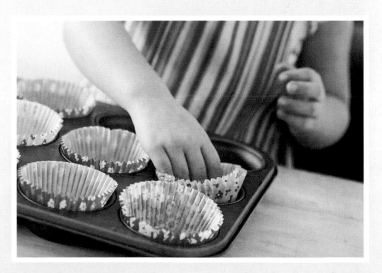

lemon, orange & passion fruit curd

Makes 5 x 225 g (8 oz) jars

Preparation time 10 minutes

Cooking time 10–15 minutes

8 passion fruit

grated rind of 3 lemons and juice of
 5 lemons

grated rind and juice of 2 large oranges

300 g (10 oz) caster sugar

225 g (7½ oz) butter, cubed

5 eggs, plus 2 egg yolks

1 Halve the passion fruit and push half of the flesh through a sieve into a jug, discarding the seeds. Whisk together the passion fruit juice, the remaining passion fruit flesh and the lemon and orange rind and juice in a medium heatproof bowl.

2 Add the sugar and butter to the bowl, then set over a saucepan of gently simmering water, stirring until melted. Stir in the eggs and continue to whisk for 10–15 minutes or until the mixture has thickened to the consistency of custard.

3 Pour the mixture into about 5 sterilized jars, seal tightly and store in the refrigerator for up to 2 weeks.

Tips and tricks

This is delicious served spread onto gluten-free Soda Bread (*see* page 116), or swirled into natural yogurt for a zesty dessert.

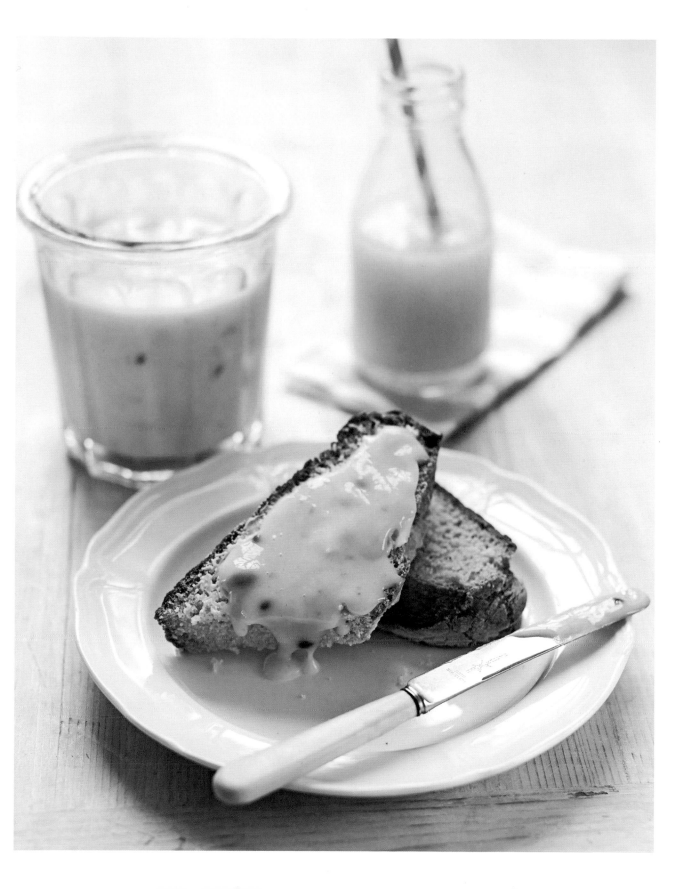

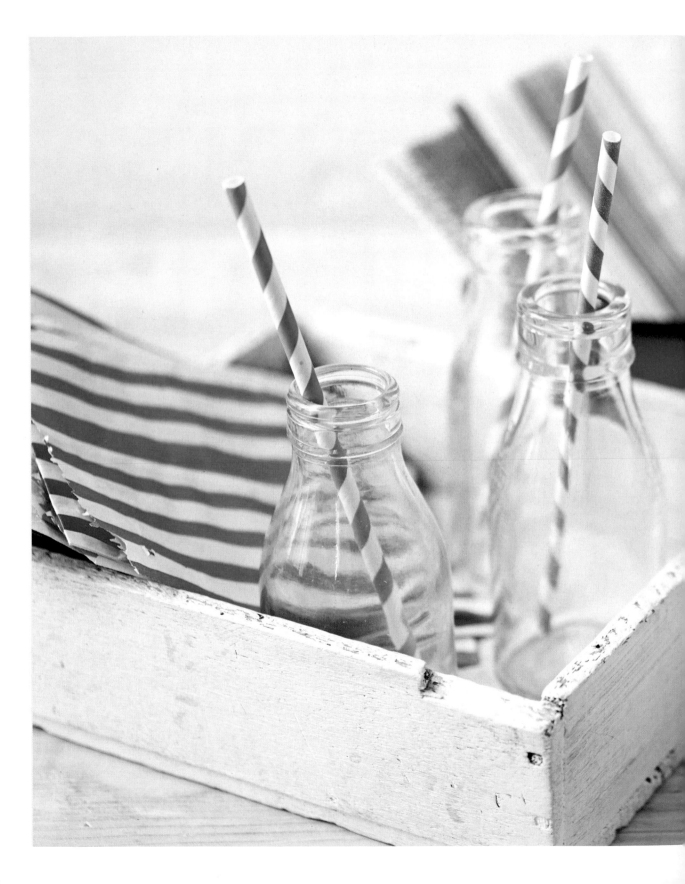

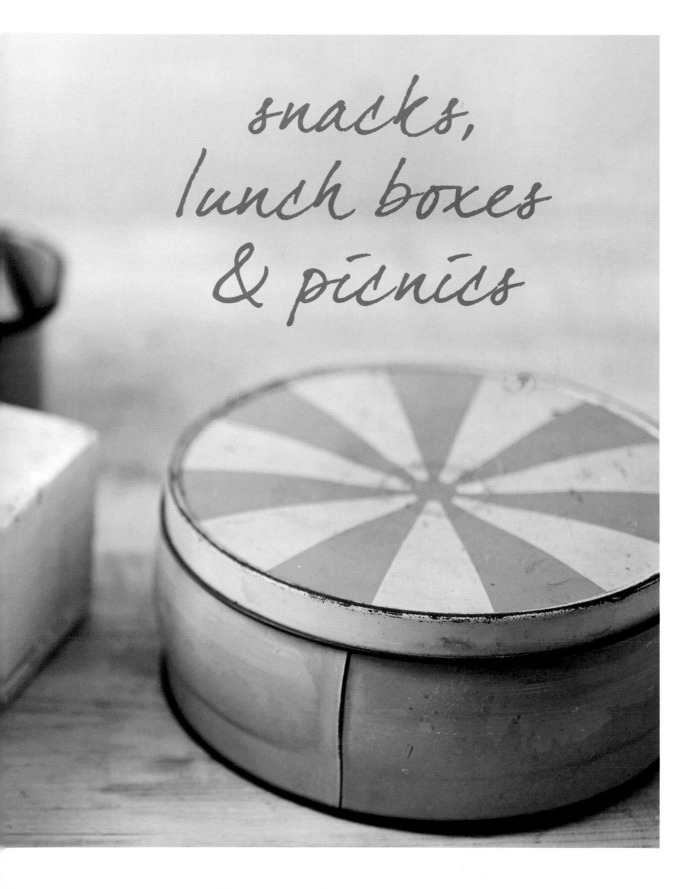

snacks,
lunch boxes
& picnics

chicken & ham soup

Serves 8

Preparation time 20 minutes

Cooking time 1 hour 20 minutes

3 tablespoons olive oil

4 large skinless chicken thighs

3 onions, chopped

2 celery sticks, sliced

375 g (12 oz) piece of lean gammon, cut
   into 1 cm (½ inch) chunks

2 bay leaves

600 ml (1 pint) gluten-free chicken stock

600 ml (1 pint) water

375 g (12 oz) potatoes, peeled and cut
   into small cubes

150 g (5 oz) frozen sweetcorn

Dumplings

125 g (4 oz) fine cornmeal

100 g (3½ oz) gluten-free flour

2 teaspoons gluten-free baking powder

1 tablespoon chopped thyme

40 g (1½ oz) cold butter

250 ml (8 fl oz) water

salt and black pepper

1 Heat the oil in a large heavy-based saucepan, add the chicken, onions and celery and fry gently for 10 minutes, stirring, until golden.

2 Add the gammon, bay leaves, stock and measurement water and bring to the boil. Reduce the heat, cover and simmer gently for 40 minutes until the chicken and ham are tender.

3 Lift out the chicken with a slotted spoon and, when cool enough to handle, shred the flesh from the bones. Return the flesh to the pan with the potatoes and sweetcorn. Simmer, covered, for 20 minutes, until the potatoes are tender.

4 Make the dumplings. Mix together the cornmeal, flour, baking powder, thyme and salt and pepper in a bowl until evenly combined. Grate the butter into the mixture and add the measurement water. Mix to a thick paste, adding a little more water if necessary.

5 Use 2 dessertspoons to roughly pat the paste into 8 rounds and spoon into the soup. Cover and simmer gently for about 10 minutes until the dumplings are light and puffy.

tomato & red pepper soup with crunchy croutons

Serves 4–6

Preparation time 10 minutes

Cooking time 20 minutes

2 tablespoons olive oil

1 onion, chopped

1 garlic clove, crushed

1 large carrot, peeled and chopped

2 red peppers, cored, deseeded and cut into chunks

handful of basil, stalks chopped and leaves torn

1 kg (2 lb) ripe tomatoes, roughly chopped

900 ml (1½ pints) gluten-free chicken or vegetable stock

100 ml (3½ fl oz) double cream

salt and black pepper

Croutons

2 thick slices of gluten-free bread, cubed

2 tablespoons grated Parmesan cheese

2 tablespoons olive oil

1 Heat the oil in a large saucepan, add the onion, garlic, carrot, red peppers and basil stalks and fry for 3–4 minutes until beginning to soften. Add the tomatoes and stock and bring to the boil, then reduce the heat and simmer for 15 minutes until the vegetables are tender.

2 Meanwhile, toss the bread cubes in the Parmesan and oil, then tip into a frying pan and cook over a medium heat until golden.

3 Transfer the vegetable mixture to a food processor or blender and whizz until smooth. Return to the pan, stir in the cream and season to taste. Reheat gently if necessary.

4 Ladle the soup into bowls, top with the torn basil and serve with the croutons.

Tips and tricks

If you prefer a heartier soup, add a can of pulses such as cannellini beans once the soup is cooked and serve topped with fried chorizo pieces.

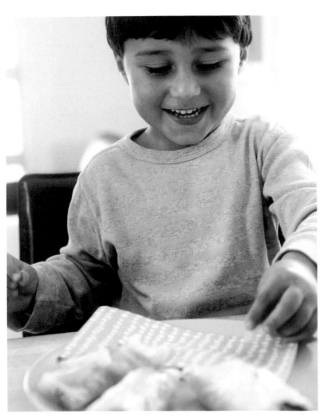
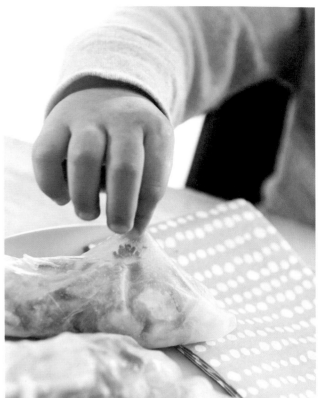
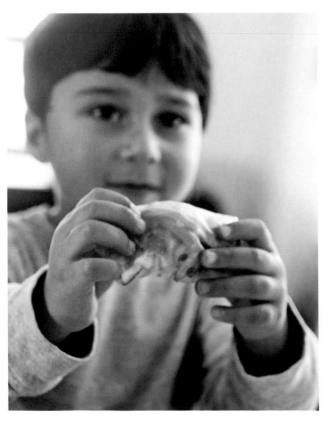
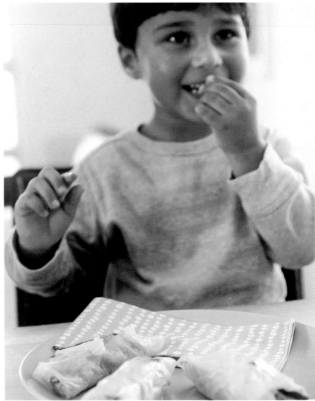

zingy prawn wraps

Makes 12

Preparation time 15 minutes

12 rice wrappers

150 g (5 oz) cooked peeled prawns, shredded

1 carrot, peeled and cut into very fine matchsticks

¼ cucumber, cut into very fine matchsticks

1 small bunch of fresh coriander, chopped

8 mint leaves, chopped

½ mango, peeled and cut into small strips

1 teaspoon sesame oil

1 teaspoon lime juice

handful of peanuts, roughly chopped (optional)

½ red chilli, deseeded and finely chopped (optional)

These wraps are a great way to introduce kids to some fresh, Asian-inspired flavours.

1 Prepare the rice wrappers according to the packet instructions.

2 Toss together all the remaining ingredients in a bowl. Divide the mixture evenly among the wrappers and roll up, ensuring the ends are tucked in. Serve straight away.

cheese & onion pancakes

Makes 4

Preparation time 15 minutes

Cooking time 10 minutes

50 g (2 oz) gram flour

50 g (2 oz) rice flour

½ teaspoon xanthan gum

3 tablespoons olive oil

200 ml (7 fl oz) water

handful of fresh coriander, chopped

½ chilli, deseeded and finely chopped (optional)

1 garlic clove, finely sliced

a little oil, for frying

100 g (3½ oz) Red Leicester cheese, grated

2 spring onions, chopped

Feel free to omit the cheese and onion topping and replace with your preferred filling instead.

1 Place the flours and xantham gum in a bowl and make a well in the centre, then gradually add the olive oil and measurement water, stirring continuously, until it forms a fairly thick batter. Stir in the coriander, chilli, if using, and garlic.

2 Heat a little oil in a nonstick pan, pour in one-quarter of the batter and tilt the pan to form a thin layer. Cook for about 1 minute until golden, then turn the pancake over and cook on the other side until golden.

3 Sprinkle over one-quarter of the cheese and spring onions, then place under a preheated hot grill and cook until the cheese has melted. Serve immediately.

4 Repeat with the remaining batter and ingredients to make the 3 remaining pancakes.

gruyère & olive drop scones

Serves 4

Preparation time 10 minutes

Cooking time 6–12 minutes

250 g (8 oz) ricotta cheese

150 ml (¼ pint) milk

3 eggs, separated

100 g (3½ oz) rice flour

1 teaspoon gluten-free baking powder

1 tablespoon chopped chives

12 pitted olives, quartered

50 g (2 oz) Gruyère cheese, grated

2 tablespoons grated Parmesan cheese

15 g (½ oz) butter

To serve (optional)

grilled bacon rashers

cherry tomatoes, halved

1 Beat together the ricotta, milk and egg yolks in a large bowl. Sift together the flour and baking powder in a separate bowl, then fold into the ricotta mixture.

2 Whisk the egg whites in a clean bowl until they form stiff peaks, then fold into the ricotta mixture with the chives, olives, Gruyère and Parmesan.

3 Heat a little of the butter in a nonstick frying pan, add spoonfuls of the mixture and fry for 1–2 minutes on each side. Transfer to a serving plate and keep warm while you cook the remaining mixture, adding the remaining butter to the pan as necessary.

4 Serve warm with crispy grilled bacon and halved cherry tomatoes, if liked.

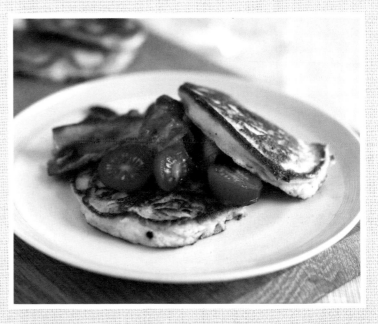

cheesy veggie pasties

Makes 4

Preparation time 15 minutes

Cooking time 50 minutes

1 leek, trimmed, cleaned and finely sliced

1 potato, cut into small cubes

100 g (3½ oz) swede, cut into small cubes

100 g 3½ oz) Caerphilly cheese, crumbled

milk, for brushing

salt and black pepper

Pastry

300 g (10 oz) rice flour, plus extra for
  dusting

½ teaspoon xanthan gum

4 tablespoons fine polenta

pinch of paprika (optional)

150 g (5 oz) cold butter, cubed

1 egg yolk

1 Make the pastry. Place the flour, xanthan gum, polenta, paprika, if using, and butter in a food processor and whizz until the mixture resembles fine breadcrumbs. Alternatively, mix together the dry ingredients in a large bowl, then add the butter and rub in with the fingertips until the mixture resembles fine breadcrumbs. Add the egg yolk and enough cold water to form a dough.

2 Meanwhile, mix together the vegetables and cheese in a bowl and season with salt and pepper.

3 Turn the pastry out on a surface lightly dusted with rice flour and divide into 4 equal-sized pieces. Gently roll each piece out to a round about 20 cm (8 inches) in diameter. Divide the vegetable mixture evenly among the pastry rounds, then close up the edges and crimp together. Make a small slit in the top of each pasty and brush with milk.

4 Transfer the pasties to a baking sheet and place in a preheated oven, 220°C (425°F), Gas Mark 7, for 10 minutes, then reduce the heat to 180°C (350°F), Gas Mark 4 and cook for a further 40 minutes until golden.

Tips and tricks

If you prefer smaller pasties, divide the pastry into 8 pieces and roll out to 15 cm (6 inches) in diameter. After the initial 10 minutes cooking, they will take only a further 25–30 minutes to bake.

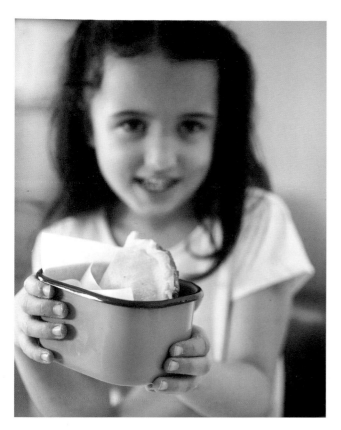
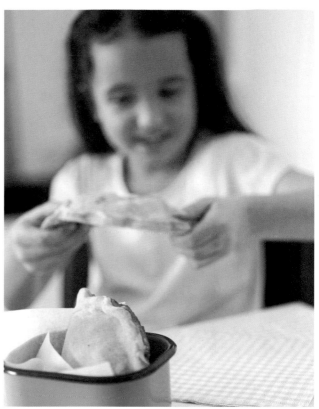
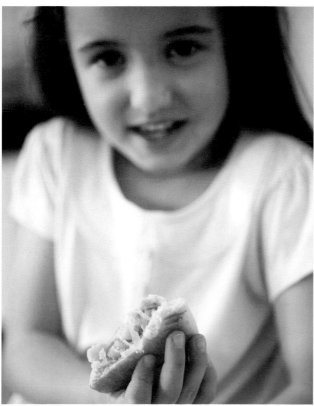
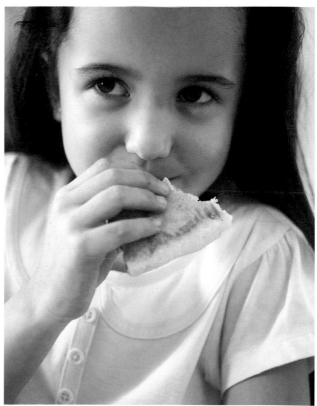

perfect beef pasties

Makes 4

Preparation time 15 minutes

Cooking time 50 minutes

200 g (7 oz) beef skirt, cut into small
  pieces

1 onion, finely chopped

1 potato, cut into small cubes

100 g (3½ oz) swede, cut into small cubes

milk, for brushing

salt and black pepper

Pastry

300 g (10 oz) rice flour, plus extra for
  dusting

½ teaspoon xanthan gum

4 tablespoons fine polenta

pinch of paprika (optional)

150 g (5 oz) cold butter, cubed

1 egg yolk

1 Make the pastry. Place the flour, xanthan gum, polenta, paprika, if using, and butter in a food processor and whizz until the mixture resembles fine breadcrumbs. Alternatively, mix together the dry ingredients in a large bowl, then add the butter and rub in with the fingertips until the mixture resembles fine breadcrumbs. Add the egg yolk and enough cold water to form a ball of dough.

2 Mix together the beef and vegetables in a bowl and season with salt and pepper.

3 Turn the pastry out on a surface lightly dusted with rice flour and divide into 4 equal-sized pieces. Gently roll each piece out to a round about 20 cm (8 inches) in diameter. Divide the beef mixture evenly among the pastry rounds, then close up the edges and crimp together. Make a small slit in the top of each pasty and brush with milk.

4 Transfer the pasties to a baking sheet and place in a preheated oven, 220°C (425°F), Gas Mark 7, for 10 minutes, then reduce the heat to 180°C (350°F), Gas Mark 4, and cook for a further 40 minutes until golden and cooked through.

Tips and tricks

If you prefer smaller pasties, divide the pastry into 8 pieces and roll out to 15 cm (6 inches) in diameter. After the initial 10 minutes cooking, they will take only a further 25–30 minutes to bake.

scotch eggs

Makes 12

Preparation time 15 minutes, plus chilling

Cooking time 15 minutes

12 quails' eggs

75 g (3 oz) gluten-free cornflakes

50 g (2 oz) fine polenta

300 g (10 oz) gluten-free sausages, skins removed, or sausagemeat

1 tablespoon chopped parsley

1 tablespoon snipped chives

good grating of nutmeg

50 g (2 oz) rice flour, plus extra for shaping into balls

2 eggs, beaten

1 litre (2¼ pints) oil, for deep-frying

salt and black pepper

These are perfect little snacks or great on a picnic.

1 Place the quails' eggs in a small saucepan, pour over boiling water and cook for 2 minutes. Drain, then transfer to a bowl of ice cold water and leave to cool.

2 Meanwhile, place the cornflakes in a food processor and whizz to fine crumbs. Tip into a shallow dish and stir in the polenta. Set aside.

3 Place the sausagemeat, herbs and nutmeg in a bowl and mash together. Season well. Divide the mixture into 12 equal-sized pieces, then roll into balls with floured hands and flatten slightly.

4 Shell the eggs, then place each one in the centre of a sausagemeat round. Gently bring the edges together to encase the eggs.

5 Place the rice flour on a plate and the beaten eggs in shallow bowl. Roll each sausagemeat ball in the flour, then dip into the beaten egg and roll in the cornflake mixture. Transfer to a plate and chill for 30 minutes.

6 Half-fill a large saucepan with oil and heat to180–190°C (350–375°F), or until a cube of bread browns in 30 seconds. Deep-fry the scotch eggs, in batches, for about 5–6 minutes minutes until golden and cooked through. Remove with a slotted spoon and retain for future use. Drain the scotch eggs on kitchen paper and serve cool.

cheesy veggie scones

Makes 8

Preparation time 10 minutes

Cooking time 12–15 minutes

175 g (6 oz) rice flour, plus extra for dusting

75 g (3 oz) cornflour

1 teaspoon gluten-free baking powder

1 teaspoon bicarbonate of soda

75 g (3 oz) cold butter, cubed, plus extra to serve

100 g (3½ oz) frozen leaf spinach, defrosted, squeezed of any liquid and chopped

4 sun-dried tomatoes in oil, drained and finely chopped

50 g (2 oz) Parmesan cheese, grated

good grating of nutmeg

1 large egg, beaten

3 tablespoons buttermilk, plus extra for brushing

1 Place the rice flour, cornflour, baking powder, bicarbonate of soda and butter in a food processor and whizz until the mixture resembles fine breadcrumbs. Alternatively, mix together the dry ingredients in a large bowl. Add the butter and rub in with the fingertips until the mixture resembles fine breadcrumbs. Mix in the spinach, sun-dried tomatoes, Parmesan and nutmeg.

2 Whisk together the egg and buttermilk in a separate bowl, stir in the flour mixture and combine to form a soft dough.

3 Turn the dough out on a surface lightly dusted with rice flour, press out to 2.5 cm (1 inch) thick and stamp out 8 scones using a 5 cm (2 inch) cutter, rerolling the trimmings as necessary.

4 Transfer to a baking sheet lightly dusted with rice flour, brush with a little buttermilk and place in a preheated oven, 220°C (425°F), Gas Mark 7, for 12–15 minutes until risen and golden. Serve warm, spread with butter.

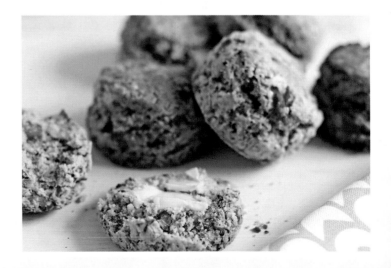

falafel with zingy salsa

Makes 12

Preparation time 10 minutes, plus chilling

Cooking time 20 minutes

400 g (13 oz) can chickpeas, rinsed and
   drained

1 small red onion, roughly chopped

1 teaspoon ground cumin

1 teaspoon ground coriander

1 teaspoon chilli powder

2 garlic cloves, crushed

handful of fresh herbs, such as mint,
   coriander and parsley

1 tablespoon gram flour

a little oil, for brushing

For the salsa

2 large tomatoes, finely chopped

½ red onion, finely sliced

½ red chilli, finely chopped

handful fresh coriander

good squeeze fresh lime

1 Place all the ingredients except the oil in a food processor or blender and blitz until well combined, but still retaining some texture.

2 Shape the mixture into 12 equal-sized smallish balls and flatten slightly. Chill until firm, about 20 minutes.

3 Transfer the falafel to a baking sheet and brush with a little oil. Place in a preheated oven, 200°C/400°F/Gas Mark 6 for 20 minutes until crisp and golden.

4 Stir together the salsa and ingredients and serve with the falafel.

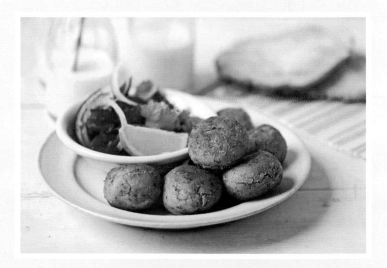

sesame pitta breads

Makes 8

Preparation time 10 minutes, plus proving

Cooking time 10 minutes

200 g (7 oz) gram flour

300 g (10 oz) rice flour, plus extra for dusting

2 teaspoons xanthan gum

50 g (1¾ oz) sesame seeds

2 teaspoons baking powder

1 tablespoon caster sugar

3 tablespoons olive oil, plus extra for oiling

300 ml (½ pint) warm milk

1 Mix the dry ingredients in a large bowl. Whisk together the oil and milk and gradually pour into the dry ingredients to form a slightly sticky dough, adding a little more flour or liquid if necessary.

2 Turn the dough out on a surface lightly dusted with rice flour and knead for 5 minutes until smooth. Place in a lightly oiled bowl, cover with a clean damp tea towel and leave in a warm place for about 1 hour to rise a little.

3 Turn the dough out on the floured surface and divide into 8 equal-sized pieces. Roll each piece out to about 0.5 cm (¼ inch) thick and flatten into a pitta shape.

4 Transfer the pittas to a wire rack, splash with a little water and place in a preheated oven, 225°C (425°F), Gas Mark 7, for 8–10 minutes until beginning to turn golden. Serve immediately.

red pepper hummus

Serves 4

Preparation time 5 minutes

280 g (10 oz) jar red peppers in oil, drained

400 g (13 oz) can chickpeas, drained

1 garlic clove, crushed

juice of ½ lemon

4 tablespoons natural yogurt

handful of fresh coriander, chopped

pinch each of cayenne pepper and salt

1 Place all the ingredients in a food processor or blender and whizz together until blended.

2 Serve with pitta breads (*see* above).

pitta crisps

Serves 8

Preparation time 5 minutes

Cooking time 8–10 minutes

8 gluten-free pitta breads (for homemade, *see* opposite)

4 tablespoons olive oil

4 garlic cloves, finely sliced

large rosemary sprig, roughly crumbled

sprinkling of sea salt

1 Cut the pittas into rough triangles. Drizzle over the oil, scatter over the garlic, rosemary and sea salt and toss to coat well.

2 Spread out the bread on a baking sheet and place in a preheated oven, 200°C (400°F), Gas Mark 6, for 8–10 minutes, turning occasionally, until crisp and golden.

cheesy dip

Serves 4

Preparation time 5 minutes

200 g (7 oz) cream cheese

2 spring onions, sliced

100 g (3½ oz) Cheddar cheese, grated

a little milk

1 Beat together all the ingredients in a bowl, adding enough milk to make a good dipping consistency.

2 Serve with fresh carrot and cucumber sticks.

feta, mint & pea dip

Preparation time 5 minutes

Cooking time 3 minutes

6 mint leaves

250 g (8 oz) frozen peas

200 g (7 oz) feta cheese

150 g (5 oz) natural yogurt

1 Put the mint and peas in a saucepan of boiling water, bring back to the boil, then drain immediately and refresh under cold running water.

2 Transfer to a food processor or blender, add the feta and yogurt and whizz together until combined, but still retaining a little texture.

baked aubergine dip

Preparation time 10 minutes

Cooking time 35–45 minutes

2 aubergines

1 tablespoon olive oil

1 garlic clove, crushed

1 cm (½ inch) piece of fresh root ginger, peeled and grated

1 small green chilli, deseeded and finely chopped

2 spring onions, finely chopped

1 teaspoon cumin seeds

½ teaspoon ground coriander

1 tablespoon chopped fresh coriander

few mint leaves, chopped

2 tablespoons natural yogurt

salt

1 Prick the aubergines all over, place on a baking sheet and bake in a preheated oven, 180°C (350°F), Gas Mark 4, for 30–40 minutes until tender.

2 Meanwhile, heat the oil in a large frying pan, add the garlic, ginger, chilli and spring onions and fry for 2 minutes. Add the cumin seeds and ground coriander and continue to fry for 1 minute. Remove the pan from the heat.

3 Cut the aubergines in half and scrape out all the flesh, add to the pan and cook for 5 minutes until all the liquid has evaporated.

4 Transfer the mixture to a food processor or blender and blitz for a few seconds until almost smooth but still retaining a little texture. Stir in all the remaining ingredients and season with salt. Serve warm or at room temperature.

lazy day baked eggs

Serves 4

Preparation time 5 minutes

Cooking time 10 minutes

butter, for greasing

4 slices of ham or smoked salmon

4 eggs

4 tablespoons double cream

4 tablespoons grated Cheddar cheese

salt and black pepper

toast, to serve

So simple yet utterly delicious. You can place a layer of whatever takes your fancy in the bottom of the ramekins – blanched asparagus is delicious.

1 Grease 4 ramekins with butter, then place 1 slice of ham or smoked salmon in the bottom of each ramekin and crack an egg into each one.

2 Pour 1 tablespoon of the cream over the top of each, then sprinkle over the cheese and season well.

3 Transfer the ramekins to a baking sheet and place in a preheated oven, 200°C (400°F), Gas Mark 6, for 10 minutes until set. Serve with toast.

Tips and tricks

This can be made into a more filling meal for the grown-ups by adding two eggs and extra fillings to each ramekin.

dosa with spicy potatoes

Makes 8

Preparation time 20 minutes, plus soaking and standing

Cooking time 30 minutes

300 g (10 oz) basmati rice

100 g (3½ oz) urad dal lentils

½ teaspoon fenugreek seeds

a little oil, for frying

salt

Spicy potatoes

650 g (23 oz) potatoes, peeled and cut into bite-sized chunks

3 tablespoons sunflower oil

2 garlic cloves, crushed

1 cm (½ inch) piece of fresh root ginger, peeled and grated

1 teaspoon mustard seeds

pinch of ground cumin

pinch of ground coriander

pinch of turmeric

Yogurt sauce

150 ml (¼ pint) natural yogurt

handful of mint and fresh coriander, chopped

½ teaspoon sugar

½ green chilli, deseeded and chopped (optional)

Although the dosa-making process takes time, the results are well worth it. Remember to start to make them the night before you want to serve them.

1 Rinse the rice and lentils, then drain and tip into a large bowl. Cover with cold water and leave to soak overnight.

2 Drain the rice and lentils, tip into a food processor or blender and blitz until smooth, adding enough water to make a smooth batter. Season with salt, then cover and leave to stand for 6 hours.

3 Cook the potatoes in a saucepan of lightly salted boiling water for about 10 minutes until just tender. Drain.

4 Heat the sunflower oil in a large frying pan, add the garlic, ginger, mustard seeds and spices and fry for 1 minute, then tip in the potatoes, toss with the spice mixture and cook over a low heat for 5–6 minutes. Keep warm.

5 Mix together all the yogurt sauce ingredients in a bowl. Set aside.

6 Heat a little oil in a heavy nonstick frying pan, add 1 tablespoon of the dosa batter to the pan and spread out thinly. Cook for 1 minute, then turn the dosa over and cook for a further 20 seconds. Remove from the pan and keep warm while you cook the remaining batter.

7 Wrap the potatoes in the dosa and serve with the yogurt sauce.

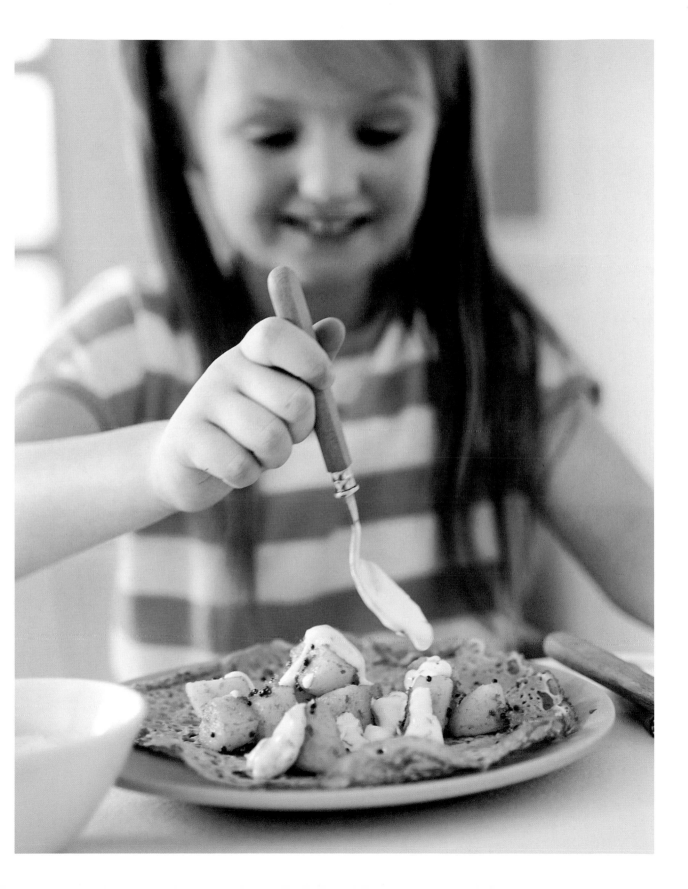

crunchy sweet potato bites

Serves 4

Preparation time 10 minutes

Cooking time 30–40 minutes

2 large sweet potatoes, ends removed and each potato cut into 6 thick slices

a little oil, for brushing

100 g (3½ oz) feta cheese, crumbled

100 g (3½ oz) mozzarella cheese, finely chopped

2 very crisp cooked bacon rashers, crumbled

2 spring onions, finely chopped

½ red or green chilli, deseeded and finely chopped

The sweet potatoes can be replaced with ordinary potatoes, if you prefer, and the toppings can be varied with whatever you have to hand. Try quartered cherry tomatoes instead of bacon for a veggie version.

1 Cook the sweet potato slices in a saucepan of boiling water for 12–15 minutes until just tender. Drain.

2 Place the slices on a baking sheet and brush both sides with a little oil. Bake in a preheated oven, 200°C (400°F) Gas Mark 6, for 10–15 minutes until beginning to crisp.

3 Mix together all the remaining ingredients in a bowl, then spoon over the potato slices. Return to the oven and cook for a further 10 minutes until golden and bubbling.

courgette, sweetcorn & mozzarella fritters

Makes 12

Preparation time 10 minutes, plus standing

Cooking time 10 minutes

2 courgettes, grated

200 g (7 oz) can sweetcorn, drained

3 spring onions, finely sliced

2 eggs, beaten

2 tablespoons gram flour

1 teaspoon gluten-free baking powder

150 g (5 oz) mozzarella cheese, diced

2 tablespoons grated Parmesan cheese

6 tablespoons olive oil

salt and black pepper

These veggie fritters are delicious served with Feta, Mint & Pea Dip (*see* page 48).

1 Sprinkle the courgettes with salt and leave to drain for about 20 minutes. Squeeze well, then transfer to a bowl, add all the remaining ingredients except the oil and mix until combined.

2 Heat the oil in a large frying pan, drop tablespoons of the fritter mixture into the pan, in batches if necessary, and fry for 1–2 minutes on each side until golden. Remove with a slotted spoon and drain on kitchen paper.

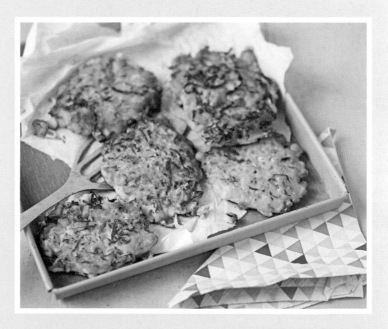

rice noodle salad

Serves 4

Preparation time 5 minutes, plus cooling

Cooking time about 5 minutes

200 g (7 oz) rice noodles

300 g (10 oz) cooked chicken, shredded

1 large carrot, peeled and grated

75 g (3 oz) mangetout, finely sliced

75 g (3 oz) bean sprouts

handful of mint and fresh coriander, chopped

Dressing

2 tablespoons peanut butter

1 teaspoon gluten-free soy sauce

juice of ½ lime

1 tablespoon sweet chilli sauce

The beauty is that rice noodles are a great gluten-free tummy filler.

1 Cook the rice noodles according to the packet instructions, then drain and leave to cool.

2 Whisk together the dressing ingredients with 2 tablespoons of water in a small bowl.

3 Place the noodles, chicken, vegetables and herbs in a large bowl and toss together. Pour over the dressing and combine until well coated.

Tips and tricks

You can use the basis of the salad and add what you like to it – prawns or shredded duck rather than the chicken, for example. You can also vary the veggies, adding courgettes or baby sweetcorn – anything goes!

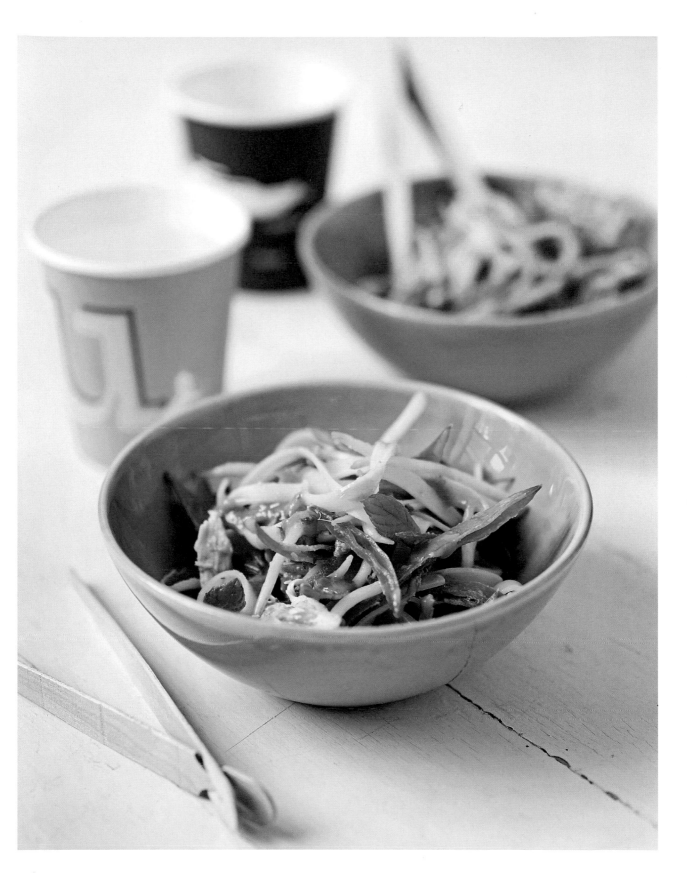

harissa-spiced chicken drumsticks

Makes 8

Preparation time 5 minutes,
  plus marinating

Cooking time 10 minutes

8 chicken drumsticks, skin removed

2 tablespoons rose harissa

6 tablespoons Greek yogurt

1 tablespoon olive oil

The drumsticks are delicious served with salad and pittas, but are also great served cold for a picnic. If you prefer, replace the harissa with tandoori paste, then prepare and cook in the same way.

1 Make 3 deep slashes in each drumstick and place in a non-metallic bowl.

2 Mix together the harissa, yogurt and oil in a bowl, then rub the mixture over the drumsticks. Cover with clingfilm and leave to marinate in the refrigerator for at least 30 minutes.

3 Transfer the drumsticks to a baking sheet and cook under a preheated hot grill for 8–10 minutes, turning occasionally, until cooked through.

ricotta & spinach tart

Serves 4

Preparation time 15 minutes, plus chilling

Cooking time 30 minutes

1 teaspoon olive oil

1 shallot, finely chopped

1 garlic clove, crushed

175 g (6 oz) baby leaf spinach

300 g (10 oz) ricotta cheese

100 g (3½ oz) light crème fraîche

4 tablespoons grated Parmesan cheese

2 eggs, lightly beaten

grating of nutmeg

salt and black pepper

Pastry

150 g (5 oz) rice flour, plus extra for dusting

100 g (3½ oz) polenta

125 g (4 oz) cold butter, cubed

25 g (1 oz) Parmesan cheese, grated

1 egg yolk

2 tablespoons milk

1 Make the pastry. Place the flour, polenta, butter and Parmesan in a food processor and whizz until the mixture resembles fine breadcrumbs. Alternatively, mix together the rice flour and polenta in a bowl. Add the butter and rub in with fingertips until the mixture resembles fine breadcrumbs. Stir in the Parmesan. Mix together the egg yolk and milk in a separate bowl and add enough to the dry ingredients to form a soft but not sticky dough. Wrap in clingfilm and chill for 30 minutes.

2 Roll the pastry out on a surface lightly dusted with rice flour and use to line a 20 cm (8 inch) fluted tart tin. Prick the base with a fork and place in a preheated oven, 200°C (400°F), Gas Mark 6, for 10 minutes. Remove from the oven.

3 Meanwhile, heat the oil in a frying pan, add the shallot and garlic and fry for 2–3 minutes until softened. Add the spinach and cook for 3–4 minutes until wilted and any moisture has evaporated.

4 Beat together the ricotta, crème fraîche, half the Parmesan and the eggs in a bowl, then season well with nutmeg and salt and pepper. Stir in the spinach and pour into the tart case, sprinkle over the remaining Parmesan and return to the oven for 20 minutes until firm and golden.

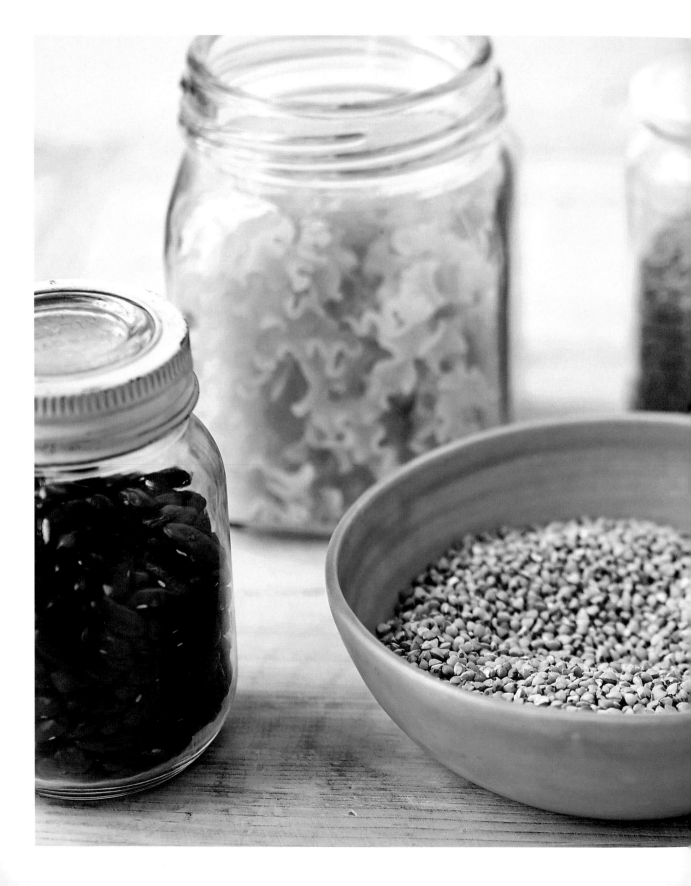

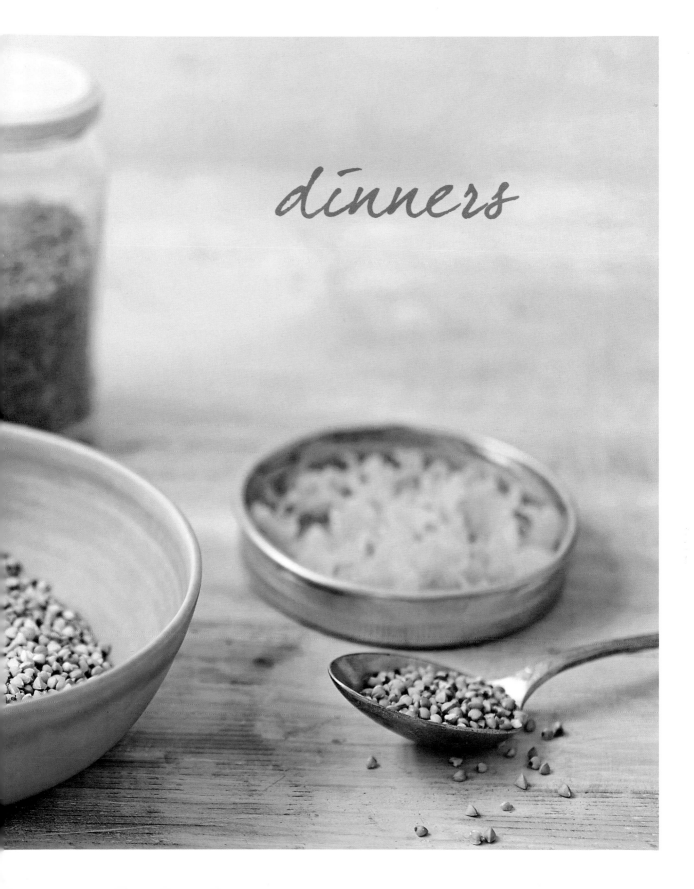

dinners

chicken & leek gratin

Serves 4

Preparation time 15 minutes

Cooking time 40–45 minutes

1 tablespoon olive oil

1 onion, chopped

1 garlic clove, crushed

4 leeks, trimmed, cleaned and chopped

4 boneless, skinless chicken breasts, about 125 g (4 oz) each, cut into chunks

1 small glass dry white wine

1 tablespoon rice flour

300 ml (½ pint) gluten-free chicken stock

150 ml (¼ pint) double cream

2 tablespoons chopped tarragon

1 tablespoon gluten-free English mustard

200 g (7 oz) fresh gluten-free breadcrumbs

100 g (3½ oz) Gruyère cheese, grated

salt and black pepper

steamed vegetables, to serve

1 Heat the oil in a large saucepan, add the onion, garlic and leeks and fry for 3–4 minutes. Transfer the vegetables to a plate, add the chicken to the pan and fry for 3 minutes until beginning to colour all over.

2 Add the wine and simmer until reduced by half. Add the flour and cook, stirring, for 1 minute, then gradually add the stock and cook, stirring continuously, until the sauce has thickened.

3 Stir in the leek mixture, cream, tarragon and mustard and season well. Transfer to an ovenproof dish, then sprinkle over the breadcrumbs and Gruyère.

4 Place in a preheated oven, 200°C (400°F), Gas Mark 6, for 25–30 minutes until golden and bubbling. Serve with steamed vegetables.

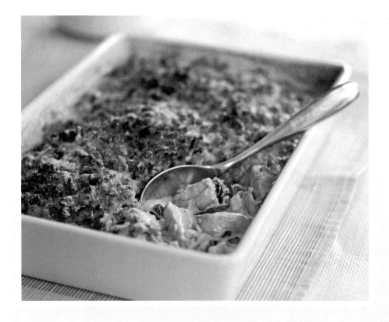

ham, leek & potato bake

Serves 4

Preparation time 15 minutes

Cooking time about 1 hour

butter, for greasing

650 g (1 lb 7 oz) potatoes, very thinly sliced

1 large leek, trimmed, cleaned and thinly sliced

150 g (5 oz) ham, chopped

2 tablespoons grated Parmesan cheese

150 ml (¼ pint) double cream

150 ml (¼ pint) gluten-free chicken or vegetable stock

150 g (5 oz) mature Cheddar cheese, grated

50g (1¾ oz) gluten-free breadcrumbs

salt and black pepper

1 Lightly butter a medium ovenproof dish or 4 individual dishes.

2 Arrange a layer of potatoes in the bottom of the dish, followed by a layer of leek and ham, then a sprinkling of Parmesan. Season well. Repeat the layers and seasoning, finishing with a layer of potatoes.

3 Stir together the cream and stock in a jug, then pour into the dish. Cover the dish with foil and place in a preheated oven, 180°C (350°F), Gas Mark 4, for 30 minutes.

4 Mix together the Cheddar and breadcrumbs in a bowl. Remove the foil from the dish and sprinkle over the potato mixture. Return to the oven and bake for a further 30–35 minutes or until golden and the potatoes are tender.

Tips and tricks

This also works well as a side dish to serve lots of people if you are feeding a crowd.

lamb & apricot meatballs with fruity salsa

Serves 4

Preparation time 10 minutes

Cooking time 10 minutes

450 g (14½ oz) minced lamb

1 garlic clove, crushed

1 teaspoon ground cumin

1 teaspoon ground coriander

few chilli flakes (optional)

25 g (1 oz) pine nuts, toasted

75 g (3 oz) ready-to-eat dried apricots, finely chopped

gluten-free Pitta Breads (*see* page 46) or steamed rice, to serve

Fruity salsa

½ mango, peeled and cut into small chunks

1 tablespoon chopped mint

1 tablespoon chopped fresh coriander

¼ cucumber, finely chopped

juice of ½ lime

1 Place the lamb, garlic, spices, pine nuts and apricots in a bowl and mix together until well combined. Shape the mixture into 20 equal-sized balls.

2 Place the meatballs on a baking tray and cook under a preheated medium grill for 6–7 minutes, turning occasionally, until browned and cooked through.

3 Meanwhile, mix together all the salsa ingredients in a bowl.

4 Serve the meatballs with the salsa and pitta breads or rice.

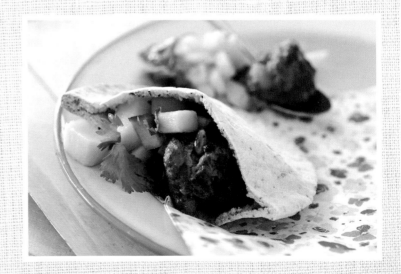

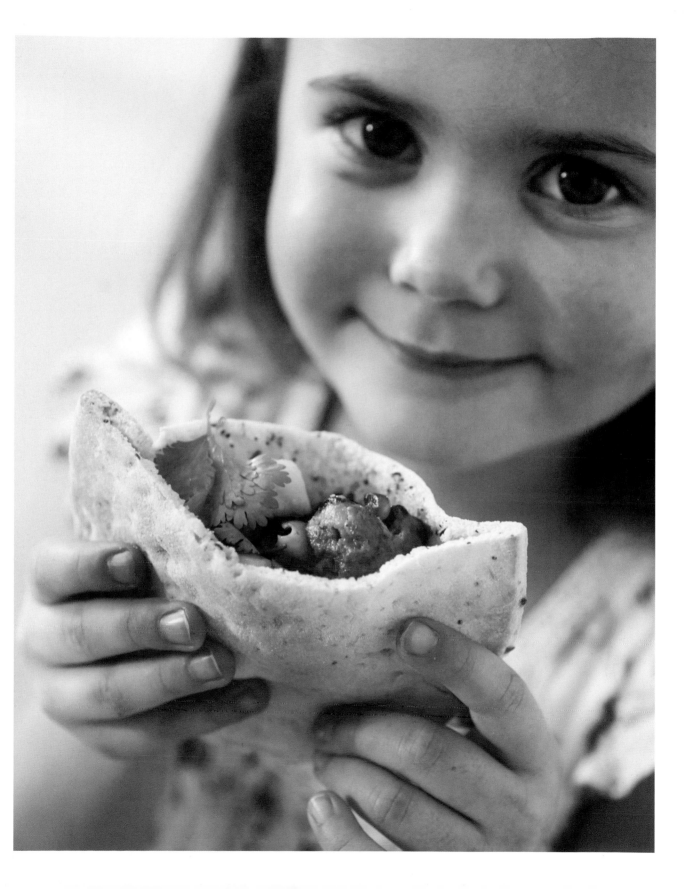

fruity mince with butternut squash

Serves 4

Preparation time 5 minutes

Cooking time 20 minutes

300 g (10 oz) butternut squash, peeled and cut into small chunks

100 g (3½ oz) green beans, trimmed and halved

1 small onion, finely chopped

300 g (10 oz) minced pork

400 g (13 oz) can chopped tomatoes

2 tablespoons tomato purée

100 g (3½ oz) ready-to-eat dried apricots, chopped

1 tablespoon chopped mixed fresh herbs, such as coriander, mint and parsley

100 ml (3½ fl oz) gluten-free chicken stock

black pepper

salt

steamed rice, to serve

1 Cook the squash and beans in a small saucepan of boiling water for 5 minutes. Drain.

2 Meanwhile, dry-fry the onion and mince in a nonstick saucepan for 4–5 minutes until the mince is browned.

3 Add all the remaining ingredients to the pan with the squash and beans and bring to the boil. Reduce the heat and simmer for 20 minutes. Season well with pepper and serve with steamed rice.

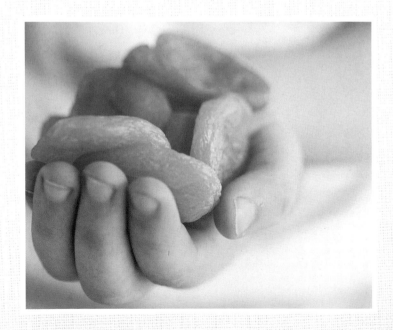

spiced lamb pie with sweet potato topping

Serves 4

Preparation time 10 minutes

Cooking time 50–55 minutes

1 tablespoon olive oil

1 onion, chopped

1 garlic clove, crushed

600 g (1¼ lb) minced lamb

1 teaspoon ground cumin

1 teaspoon ground coriander

pinch of ground cinnamon

400 g (13 oz) can chopped tomatoes

1 tablespoon tomato purée

150 ml (¼ pint) gluten-free beef or
  vegetable stock

Topping

650 g (1 lb 7 oz) sweet potatoes, peeled
  and chopped

1 tablespoon chopped fresh coriander

6 tablespoons Greek yogurt

1 tablespoon butter

salt and black pepper

1 Heat the oil in a large saucepan or flameproof casserole, add the onion and garlic and fry for 2–3 minutes until softened. Add the mince and fry until browned, then add the spices and cook for a further 1 minute.

2 Add the tomatoes, purée and stock and bring to the boil, then reduce the heat, cover and simmer for 45 minutes until thickened slightly and the mince is tender.

3 Meanwhile, cook the sweet potatoes in a saucepan of lightly salted boiling water for 15–20 minutes until tender. Drain, then season well and mash together with the coriander, Greek yogurt and butter.

4 Transfer the lamb mixture to a medium flameproof dish and spoon over the sweet potato mash. Cook under a preheated hot grill for 2–3 minutes until golden and bubbling.

beef pies with pesto pastry

Serves 4

Preparation time 15 minutes, plus chilling

Cooking time 2½–3 hours

2 tablespoons cornflour

650 g (1 lb 7 oz) lean stewing steak, cubed

2 tablespoons sunflower oil

1 large onion, sliced

1 large carrot, peeled and chopped

1 thyme sprig

450 ml (¾ pint) gluten-free beef stock

milk, for brushing

salt and black pepper

Pastry

200 g (7 oz) rice flour

3 tablespoons fine polenta

pinch of paprika (optional)

100 g (3½ oz) cold butter, cubed

1 tablespoon pesto

1 egg yolk

1 egg, beaten, to brush

Serve these pies with lots of yummy veggies.

1 Place the cornflour on a plate and season with salt and pepper. Add the steak pieces and toss in the flour until coated.

2 Heat half the oil in a heavy-based flameproof casserole, add the onion, carrot and thyme and fry for 3–4 minutes until the vegetables begin to soften. Remove from the pan and set aside.

3 Add the steak to the pan and brown on all sides. Return the vegetables to the pan and stir in the stock. Bring to the boil, then reduce the heat, cover and simmer for 1½–2 hours or until the meat is tender.

4 Meanwhile, make the pastry. Place flour, polenta, paprika and butter in a food processor and whizz until the mixture resembles fine breadcrumbs. Alternatively, mix together the dry ingredients in a large bowl. Add the butter and rub in with the fingertips until the mixture resembles fine breadcrumbs. Beat together the pesto and egg yolk in a separate bowl and stir into the flour mixture with enough cold water to form a dough.

5 Fill 4 individual ovenproof pie dishes with the steak mixture. Roll the pastry out between 2 sheets of clingfilm to 0.5 cm (¼ inch) thick, then cut out rounds, big enough to cover your particular dishes. Moisten the edges of the pie dishes and use the pastry rounds to top the pie dishes. Brush the tops with a little egg, then place in a preheated oven, 180°C (350°F), Gas Mark 4, for 35–40 minutes until the pastry is cooked through and golden.

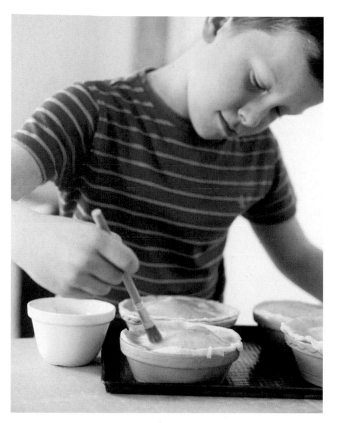
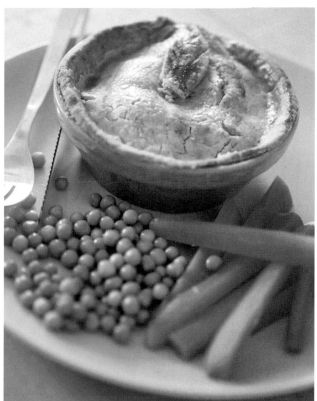
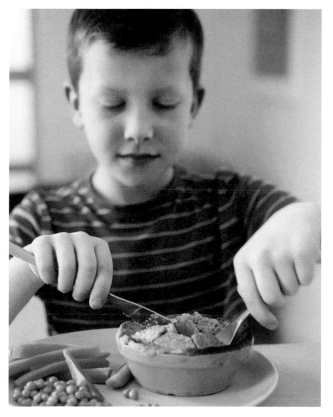
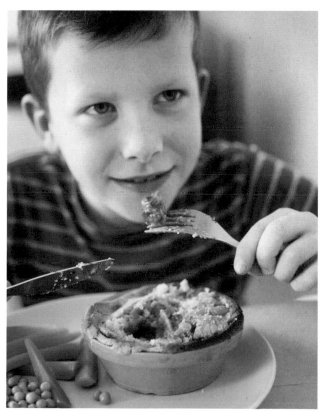

aubergine parmigiana

Serves 4

Preparation time 10 minutes

Cooking time 40–45 minutes

2 large aubergines, sliced

2 tablespoons olive oil

150 g (5 oz) mozzarella cheese, roughly chopped

4 tablespoons grated Parmesan cheese

salt and black pepper

Tomato sauce

1 tablespoon olive oil

1 garlic clove, crushed

1 small onion, finely chopped

400 g (13 oz) can plum tomatoes

handful of basil, torn

To serve

salad

crusty gluten-free bread

1 Make the tomato sauce. Heat the oil in a saucepan, add the garlic and onion and fry for 3–4 minutes until softened. Add the tomatoes and basil and bring to the boil, then reduce the heat and simmer for 15 minutes.

2 Meanwhile, brush the aubergine slices on each side with the oil. Heat a griddle until hot and cook the aubergine slices for 1–2 minutes on each side until tender and browned.

3 Spoon a little of the tomato sauce into an ovenproof dish, layer over half the aubergines, scatter over half the mozzarella and Parmesan and season well. Repeat the layering with the remaining ingredients, finishing with a scattering of the cheeses.

4 Place in a preheated oven, 200°C (400°F), Gas Mark 6, for 20–25 minutes until golden. Serve with salad and crusty bread.

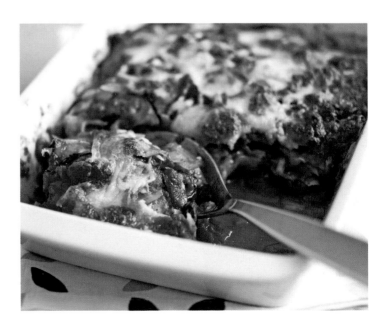

potato pizza margherita

Serves 3–4

Preparation time 20 minutes, plus cooling

Cooking time 45 minutes

1 kg (2 lb) baking potatoes, peeled and cut into small chunks

3 tablespoons olive oil, plus extra for oiling

1 egg, beaten

50 g (2 oz) Parmesan or Cheddar cheese, grated

4 tablespoons gluten-free sun-dried tomato paste or tomato ketchup

500 g (1 lb) small tomatoes, thinly sliced

125 g (4 oz) mozzarella cheese, thinly sliced

1 tablespoon chopped thyme, plus extra sprigs to garnish (optional)

salt

1 Boil the potatoes in salted water for 15 minutes or until tender. Drain well, return to the pan and cool for 10 minutes.

2 Add 2 tablespoons of the oil, the egg and half the cheese to the potato and mix well. Turn out on to an oiled baking sheet and spread out to form a 25 cm (10 inch) round. Place in a preheated oven, 200°C (400°F), Gas Mark 6, for 15 minutes.

3 Remove from the oven and spread with the tomato paste or ketchup. Arrange the tomato and mozzarella slices on top. Scatter with the remaining grated Parmesan, thyme, if using, and a little salt. Drizzle with the remaining oil.

4 Return to the oven for a further 15 minutes until the potato is crisp around the edges and the cheese is melting. Cut into generous wedges, garnish with thyme sprigs, if liked, and serve.

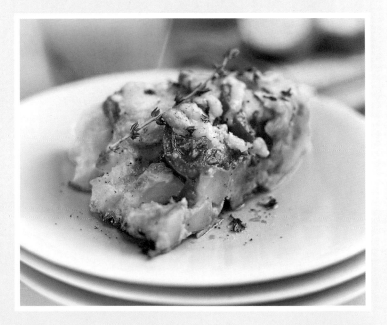

golden buttermilk chicken & zingy coleslaw

Serves 6

Preparation time 10 minutes, plus marinating

Cooking time 25–30 minutes

12 chicken drumsticks or boneless chicken thighs

140 ml (¼ pint) buttermilk

good pinch of cayenne pepper

75 g (3 oz) rice flour

100 g (3½ oz) gram flour

pinch of chilli powder

pinch of dried oregano

4 tablespoons sunflower oil, for frying

salt

Coleslaw

½ red or white cabbage, finely sliced

1 large carrot, peeled and cut into ribbons

2 spring onions, finely sliced

juice of 1 lime

150 ml (¼ pint) natural yogurt

1 Place the chicken pieces in a non-metallic bowl. Stir together the buttermilk and cayenne in a jug and season well. Pour over the chicken and toss well to coat, then cover and leave to marinate in the refrigerator for at least 1 hour, and preferably overnight.

2 Mix together the flours, chilli powder and oregano in a bowl and tip on to a plate. Remove the chicken from the marinade, draining off any excess buttermilk, then dust the pieces well with the flour mixture.

3 Heat the oil in a large deep frying pan to 180–190°C (350–375°F), or until a cube of bread browns in 30 seconds. Fry the chicken for 3–4 minutes on each side until golden, then transfer to a baking sheet. Place in a preheated oven, 220°C (425°F), Gas Mark 7, for 20 minutes or until cooked through.

4 Make the coleslaw. Place all the ingredients in a serving bowl and toss together, then serve with the chicken.

vegetable spaghetti bolognese

Serves 2

Preparation time 10 minutes

Cooking time 40–50 minutes

1 tablespoon vegetable oil

1 onion, finely chopped

1 garlic clove, finely chopped

1 celery stick, finely chopped

1 carrot, peeled and finely chopped

75 g (3 oz) chestnut mushrooms, roughly
chopped

1 tablespoon tomato purée

400 g (13 oz) can chopped tomatoes

250 ml (8 fl oz) red wine or gluten-free
vegetable stock

pinch of dried mixed herbs

1 teaspoon yeast extract

150 g (5 oz) textured vegetable protein

2 tablespoons chopped parsley

200 g (7 oz) gluten-free spaghetti

salt and black pepper

grated Parmesan cheese, to serve

1 Heat the oil in a large heavy-based saucepan over a medium heat. Add the onion, garlic, celery, carrot and mushrooms and cook, stirring frequently, for 5 minutes or until softened. Add the tomato purée and cook, stirring, for a further minute.

2 Add the tomatoes, wine or stock, herbs, yeast extract and TVP. Bring to the boil, then reduce the heat, cover and simmer for 30–40 minutes until the vegetable protein is tender. Stir in the parsley and season well.

3 Meanwhile, cook the pasta in a large saucepan of salted boiling water according to the packet instructions until al dente. Drain well.

4 Divide the pasta between 2 serving plates, top with the vegetable mixture and serve immediately with a scattering of grated Parmesan.

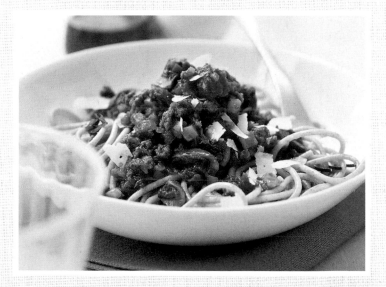

sausage & pea pasta

Serves 4

Preparation time 5 minutes

Cooking time about 10 minutes

1 tablespoon olive oil

6 gluten-free sausages, chopped

½ gluten-free chicken or vegetable stock cube

4 tablespoons boiling water

2 teaspoons gluten-free Dijon mustard

150 ml (¼ pint) double cream or light crème fraîche

300 g (10 oz) gluten-free pasta

200 g (7 oz) frozen peas

1 Heat the oil in large frying pan, add the sausages and fry for 4–5 minutes until browned all over.

2 Crumble in the stock cube and add the measurement water. Bubble and scrape all the sticky bits from the base of the pan. Stir in the mustard and cream or crème fraîche and bubble for a further few minutes.

3 Meanwhile, cook the pasta in a saucepan of boiling water according to the packet instructions until tender, adding the peas 2 minutes before the end of the cooking time. Drain and return to the pan, then toss through the sausage mixture and serve.

hazelnut, parsley & basil pesto

Serves 4

Preparation time 5 minutes

Cooking time about 10 minutes

125 g (4 oz) hazelnuts, toasted

1 garlic clove, crushed

handful each of parsley and basil leaves

100 g (3½ oz) Parmesan cheese, grated

good pinch of chilli flakes (optional)

100 ml (3½ fl oz) light olive oil

300 g (10 oz) gluten-free fusilli

1 Place all the ingredients in a food processor or blender and whizz until blitzed but still retaining a little texture.

2 Cook the fusilli in a saucepan of boiling water according to the packet instructions until tender. Stir through the pesto and serve immediately.

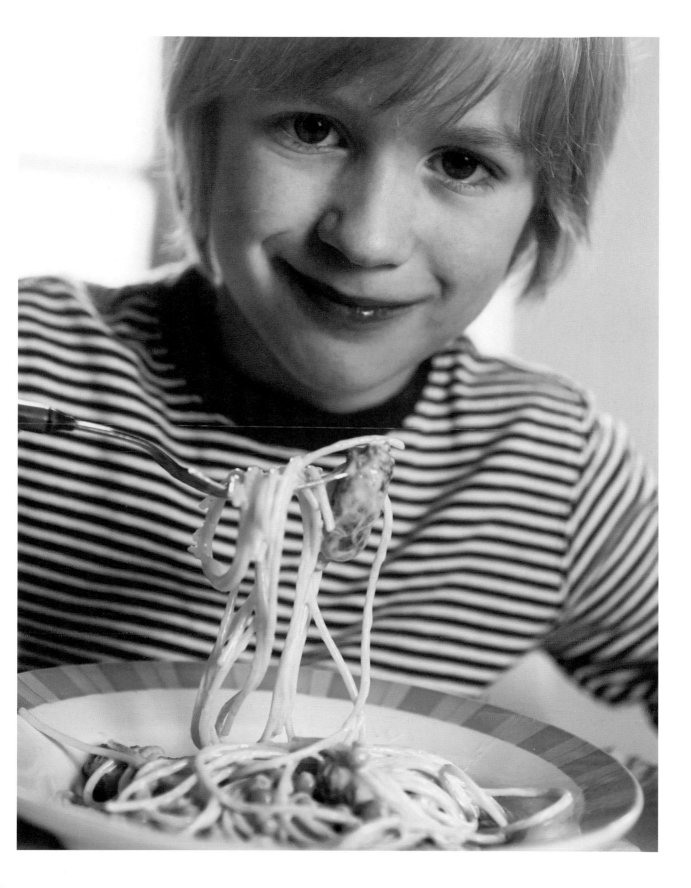

spicy chorizo & tomato sauce

Serves 4

Preparation time 5 minutes

Cooking time 15 minutes

150 g (5 oz) chorizo, chopped

1 garlic clove, crushed

400 g (13 oz) can plum tomatoes, blitzed
 in a food processor or blender until
 smooth, or 400 ml (14 fl oz) passata

handful of basil, roughly chopped

pinch of sugar

300 g (10 oz) gluten-free penne

grated Parmesan cheese, to serve

1 Dry-fry the chorizo in a medium saucepan over a medium heat until beginning to brown. Add all the remaining ingredients and bring to the boil, then reduce the heat and simmer gently for 10 minutes.

2 Cook the penne in a saucepan of boiling water according to the packet instructions until tender. Stir through the sauce and serve sprinkled with Parmesan.

courgette & mascarpone sauce

Serves 4

Preparation time 5 minutes

Cooking time 10–15 minutes

1 tablespoon olive oil

1 garlic clove, crushed

2 courgettes, coarsely grated

grated rind of 1 lemon

4 tablespoons mascarpone cheese

2 tablespoons grated Parmesan cheese

50 g (2 oz) pine nuts, toasted

300 g (10 oz) gluten-free pasta

1 Heat the oil in a frying pan, add the garlic, courgettes and lemon rind and fry gently for 3–4 minutes until softened.

2 Meanwhile, cook the pasta in a saucepan of boiling water according to the packet instructions until tender.

3 Toss the sauce through the pasta and stir in the mascarpone cheese and Parmesan. Sprinkle over the pine nuts and serve.

bacon & spinach pasta

Serves 4

Preparation time 10 minutes

Cooking time 10–15 minutes

375 g (12 oz) gluten-free pasta

1 tablespoon olive oil

200 g (7 oz) streaky bacon, sliced

1 onion, sliced

2 tablespoons pine nuts

175 g (6 oz) baby leaf spinach

300 g (10 oz) cherry tomatoes, halved

6 tablespoons single cream

2 tablespoons grated Parmesan cheese

4 spring onions, sliced

salt and black pepper

1 Cook the pasta in a saucepan of salted boiling water according to the packet instructions until tender.

2 Meanwhile, heat the oil in a frying pan, add the bacon and onion and fry for 3–4 minutes until the bacon is crisp and the onion softened.

3 Add the pine nuts and cook for 1 minute. Stir in the spinach and tomatoes and cook until the spinach is just wilted.

4 Drain the pasta and return to the pan, then stir in the spinach mixture. Mix in the cream, Parmesan and spring onions, season well and serve immediately.

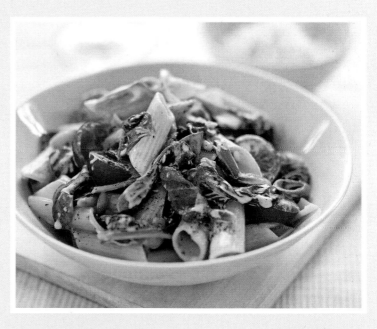

chicken & spinach curry

Serves 4

Preparation time 5 minutes

Cooking time about 20 minutes

1 tablespoon vegetable oil

4 boneless, skinless chicken breasts, about 125 g (4 oz) each, halved lengthways

1 onion, sliced

2 garlic cloves, chopped

1 green chilli, deseeded and chopped

4 cardamom pods

1 teaspoon cumin seeds

1 teaspoon chilli flakes

1 teaspoon ground coriander

1 teaspoon turmeric

1 tablespoon mild curry powder

250 g (8 oz) baby leaf spinach

300 g (10 oz) tomatoes, chopped

150 ml (¼ pint) light Greek yogurt

2 tablespoons chopped fresh coriander

steamed rice, to serve

1 Heat the oil in large nonstick saucepan or frying pan, add the chicken, onion and garlic and fry for 4–5 minutes until the chicken is beginning to brown and the onion softens. Stir in the chilli, cardamom, cumin, chilli flakes, ground coriander, turmeric and curry powder and fry for a further 1 minute.

2 Add the spinach and cook gently until wilted, then stir in the tomatoes, cover and simmer for 15 minutes, removing the lid for the final 5 minutes of cooking time.

3 Stir in the yogurt and coriander and serve with steamed rice.

Tips and tricks

Gluten-free naan breads are not very common but if you prefer to eat your curry with bread, try the gluten-free pittas on page 46, or wrapped in the dosas on page 50.

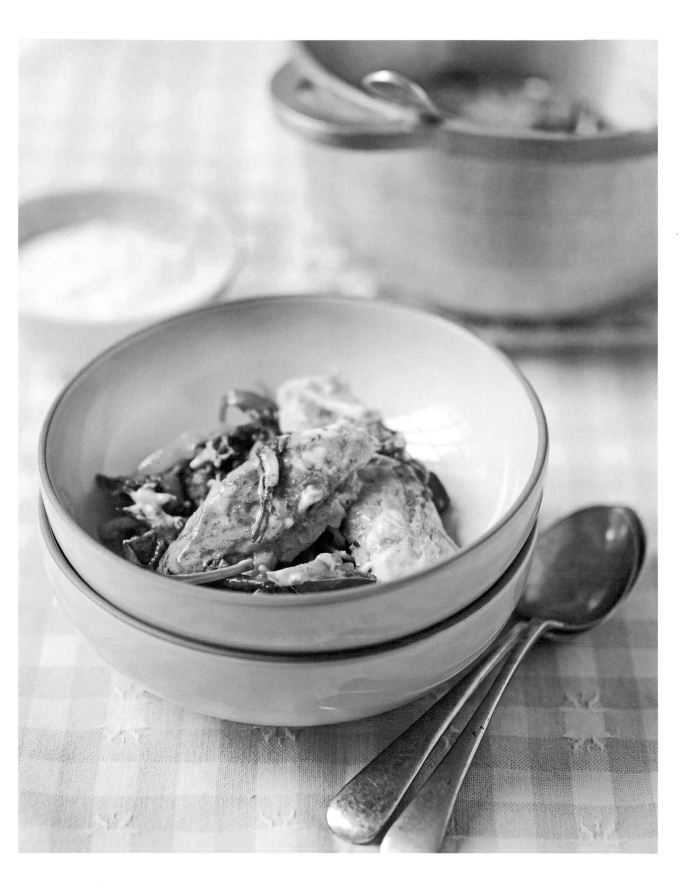

posh baked beans with poached eggs

Serves 4

Preparation time 5 minutes

Cooking time 25 minutes

1 tablespoon sunflower oil

1 onion, chopped

1 garlic clove, crushed

75 g (3 oz) bacon or chorizo, chopped

400 g (13 oz) can chopped tomatoes

1 tablespoon tomato purée

2 x 400 g (13 oz) cans cannellini beans, rinsed and drained

½ teaspoon caster sugar

1 tablespoon white wine vinegar

4 eggs

These baked beans are delicious served with toasted Cheesy Bread (*see* page 113). If you prefer a vegetarian option, omit the bacon or chorizo.

1 Heat the oil in a medium frying pan, add the onion and garlic and fry gently for 2–3 minutes until softened. Add all the remaining ingredients except the eggs, cover and simmer for 20 minutes until thickened slightly.

2 Make 4 wells in the tomato mixture and crack an egg into each, pop the lid back on and cook for 2–3 minutes until the eggs are just cooked through.

vegetable & lentil bake

Serves 4

Preparation time 10 minutes

Cooking time 50 minutes

1 red pepper, cored, deseeded and sliced

2 courgettes, halved lengthways and cut into chunks

1 large sweet potato, peeled and cut into chunks

1 red onion, cut into wedges

1 tablespoon olive oil

150 g (5 oz) red lentils

750 ml (1¼ pints) gluten-free vegetable stock

150 g (5 oz) feta cheese, crumbled

100 g (3½ oz) mozzarella cheese, chopped

2 tablespoons grated Parmesan cheese

1 Put the red pepper, courgettes, sweet potato and onion in a large roasting tin and drizzle over the oil. Place in a preheated oven, 220°C (425°F), Gas Mark 7, for 25–30 minutes until charred and softened.

2 Remove from the oven and sprinkle over the lentils, then pour over the stock. Return to the oven and bake for a further 15 minutes until the lentils are tender.

3 Mix together the cheeses in a bowl, then sprinkle over the bake and cook for a further 2–3 minutes until melted.

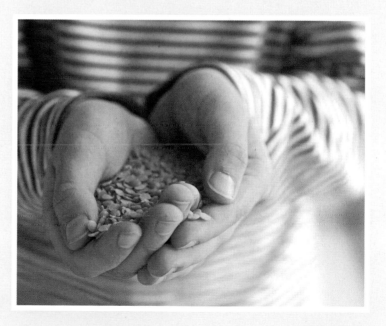

battered fish with pea purée

Serves 4

Preparation time 10 minutes

Cooking time 5 minutes

oil, for deep-frying

100 g (3½ oz) gram flour, plus extra for coating

150 ml (¼ pint) ice-cold sparkling water

4 small white fish fillets, such as haddock or whiting, about 125 g (4 oz) each

salt and black pepper

Pea purée

400 g (13 oz) frozen peas

1 small onion, finely chopped

300 ml (½ pint) boiling gluten-free vegetable stock

4 tablespoons double cream

Serve this the traditional way, with chips.

1 Half-fill a deep frying pan with oil and heat to 180–190°C (350–375°F), or until a cube of bread browns in 30 seconds.

2 Meanwhile, place the flour in a large bowl and season well. Pour in the sparkling water and whisk to combine. Dredge the fish fillets with flour, then dip into the batter.

3 Deep-fry the fish in the hot oil for 3–4 minutes, turning occasionally, until golden on all sides and cooked through.

4 Meanwhile, put the peas, onion and stock in a saucepan and simmer for 3 minutes. Drain, then transfer to a food processor or blender, add the cream and whizz to a purée. Season and serve with the battered fish.

salmon & pea risotto

Serves 4

Preparation time 5 minutes

Cooking time 25 minutes

1 teaspoon olive oil

1 small onion, finely chopped

350 g (12 oz) risotto rice

1.2 litres (2 pints) boiling gluten-free
  vegetable stock

250 g (9 oz) skinless salmon fillet, cubed

200 g (7 oz) frozen peas, defrosted

2 tablespoons chopped parsley

3 tablespoons grated Parmesan cheese

rocket and tomato salad, to serve

1 Heat the oil in a large nonstick frying pan, add the onion and fry for 2–3 minutes until beginning to soften. Add the rice and stir well to coat in the oil.

2 Add the stock a ladleful at a time, stirring continuously, until the liquid has been absorbed and the rice is just tender – about 20 minutes.

3 Add the salmon and peas with the final ladleful of stock and cook until the fish is just cooked through and the peas are tender. Stir in the parsley and Parmesan.

4 Serve the risotto with rocket and tomato salad.

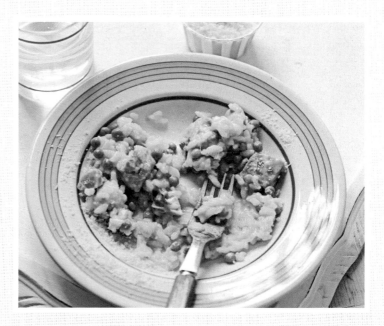

sweet potatoes with tomato salsa

Serves 4

Preparation time 10 minutes

Cooking time 45 minutes

4 large sweet potatoes, about 275 g
  (9 oz) each

2 tablespoons olive oil

100 g (3½ oz) Emmental or Cheddar
  cheese, grated

salt

green salad, to serve

Salsa

4 large tomatoes, finely chopped

1 small red onion, finely chopped

2 celery sticks, finely chopped

handful of fresh coriander, chopped

4 tablespoons lime juice

4 teaspoons caster sugar

1 Scrub the potatoes and put them in a small roasting tin. Prick with a fork, drizzle with the oil and sprinkle with a little salt. Place in a preheated oven, 200°C (400°F), Gas Mark 6, for 45 minutes until tender.

2 Meanwhile, make the salsa. Mix together the tomatoes, onion, celery, coriander, lime juice and sugar in a bowl.

3 Halve the potatoes and fluff up the flesh with a fork. Sprinkle with the cheese and top with the salsa. Serve with a green salad.

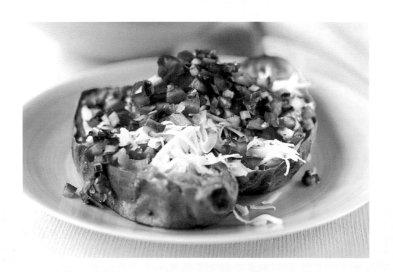

cauliflower & broccoli bake

Serves 4

Preparation time 10 minutes

Cooking time 20 minutes

8 streaky bacon rashers

50 g (2 oz) butter

1 cauliflower, cut into florets

1 head of broccoli, cut into florets

25 g (1 oz) cornflour

300 ml (½ pint) milk

100 g (3½ oz) Gruyère cheese, grated

50 g (2 oz) gluten-free fresh breadcrumbs

salt and black pepper

1 Cook the bacon rashers under a medium grill, turning once, until cooked through and crisp.

2 Meanwhile, heat half the butter in a frying pan, add the cauliflower and broccoli and fry until just tender. Transfer to an ovenproof dish.

3 Melt the remaining butter in a saucepan, add the cornflour and cook, stirring, for 1 minute. Gradually add the milk and cook, stirring continuously, until thickened and smooth, then season well. Stir in two-thirds of the Gruyère, then crumble in half the cooked bacon.

4 Pour the sauce over the vegetables. Mix together the remaining Gruyère and the breadcrumbs and sprinkle over the top with the remaining bacon.

5 Place in a preheated oven, 200°C (400°F), Gas Mark 6, for 10–12 minutes until golden and bubbling.

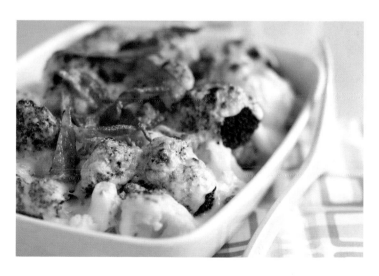

crab cakes

Serves 4

Preparation time 15 minutes, plus cooling and chilling

Cooking time 20 minutes

300 g (10 oz) potatoes, peeled and chopped

375 g (12 oz) fresh white crab meat

3 spring onions, sliced

handful of fresh coriander, leaves and stalks finely chopped

good squeeze of lime juice

½ chilli, deseeded and finely chopped

1 egg yolk

3 tablespoons polenta

2 tablespoons vegetable oil

salt and black pepper

To serve

gluten-free chilli dipping sauce

lime wedges

mixed leaf salad

1 Cook the potatoes in a saucepan of salted boiling water for 15 minutes or until tender. Drain well, return to the pan and mash. Leave to cool. Stir in all the remaining ingredients except the polenta and oil.

2 Put the polenta on a plate, shape the crab mixture into 8 cakes and coat in the polenta. Cover with clingfilm and chill for 20 minutes.

3 Heat the oil in a large frying pan, add the cakes and fry for 2–3 minutes on each side until golden.

4 Serve with a mixed leaf salad, gluten-free chilli dipping sauce and lime wedges.

spinach & fish pie

Serves 4

Preparation time 15 minutes

Cooking time 45–55 minutes

1 tablespoon olive oil

1 onion, chopped

175 g (6 oz) baby leaf spinach

50 g (2 oz) butter

25 g (1 oz) rice flour

600 ml (1 pint) milk

1 tablespoon gluten-free wholegrain
  mustard

good grating of nutmeg

650 g (1 lb 7 oz) mixed skinless salmon,
  haddock and smoked haddock fillets,
  cut into chunks

200 g (7 oz) raw prawns, peeled and
  deveined

salt and black pepper

Potato topping

1 kg (2 lb) potatoes, peeled and cut into
  chunks

knob of butter

100 ml (3½ fl oz) single cream

1 Make the potato topping. Cook the potatoes in a saucepan of salted boiling water for 15 minutes or until tender. Drain well and return to the pan. Mash together with the butter and cream and season well.

2 Heat the oil in a large saucepan, add the onion and fry for 2–3 minutes until beginning to soften. Add the spinach to the pan and cook until wilted and any liquid has evaporated.

3 Melt the butter in a saucepan, add the flour and cook, stirring, for 1 minute. Gradually add the milk and cook, stirring continuously, until thickened and smooth. Stir in the mustard and nutmeg and season well.

4 Arrange the fish and the prawns in a large ovenproof dish and top with the spinach. Pour over the sauce, spoon the mash on top and place in a preheated oven, 200°C (400°F), Gas Mark 6, for 30–35 minutes until golden and bubbling.

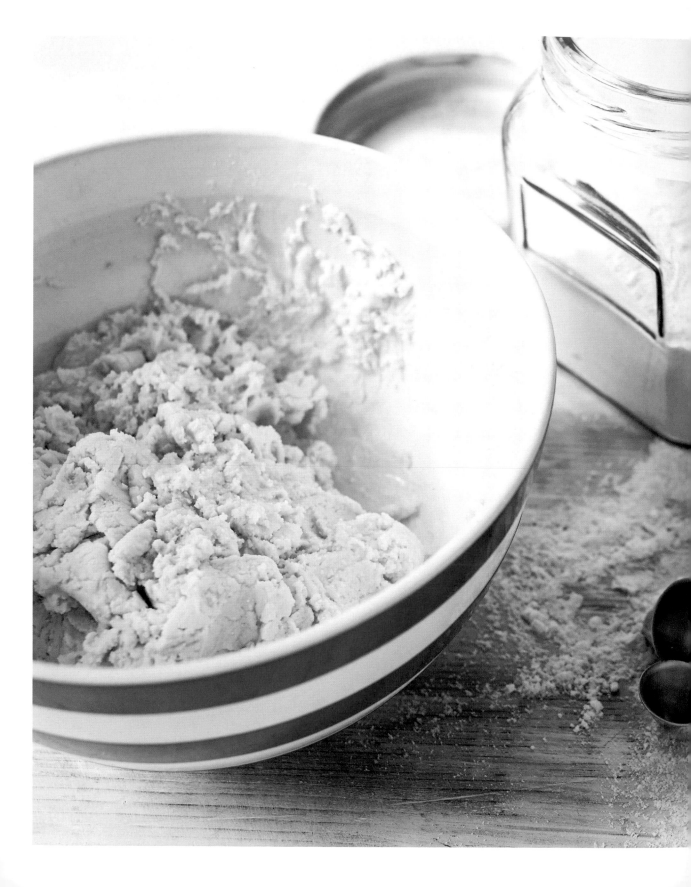

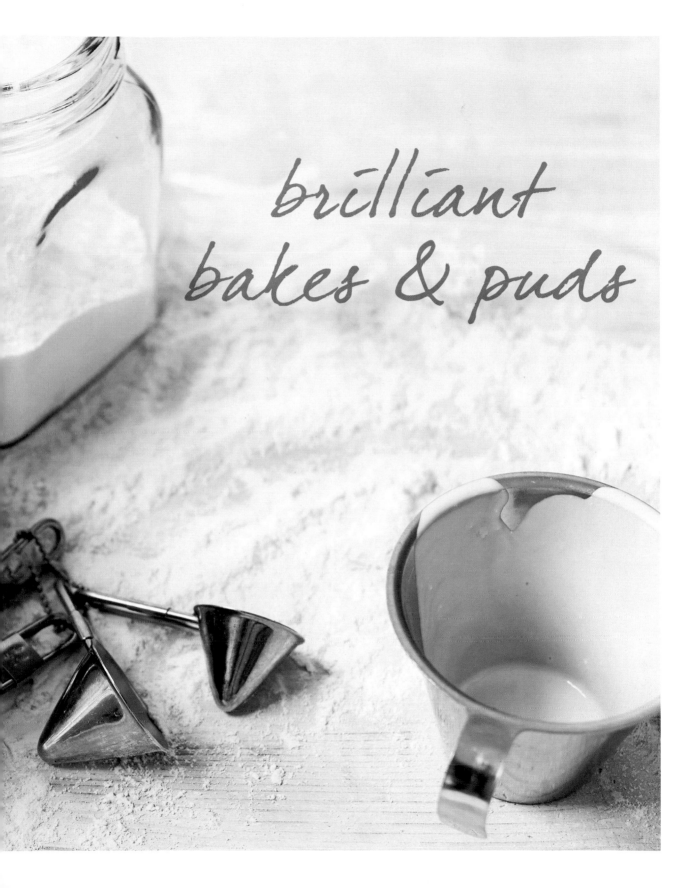

brilliant
bakes & puds

carrot & orange muffins

Makes 12

Preparation time 10 minutes

Cooking time 15–18 minutes

150 g (5 oz) golden caster sugar

150 g (5 oz) rice flour

100 g (3½ oz) cornflour

1 tablespoon gluten-free baking powder

1 carrot, peeled and grated

2 tablespoons buttermilk

150 g (5 oz) butter, melted

3 eggs, beaten

grated rind of 2 oranges

125 g (4 oz) icing sugar

1 Line a 12-hole muffin tray with muffin cases.

2 Mix together the sugar, flours, baking powder and carrot in a bowl. Whisk together the buttermilk, butter, eggs and orange rind in a jug, then pour into the dry ingredients and stir until just combined.

3 Spoon the mixture into the muffin cases and place in a preheated oven, 180°C (350°F), Gas Mark 4, for 15–18 minutes until golden and springy to the touch. Leave to cool.

4 Sift the icing sugar into a bowl. Add a tablespoon warm water and stir until the icing is thick enough to coat the spoon, adding extra drops of water as necessary. Drizzle over the muffins and leave to set.

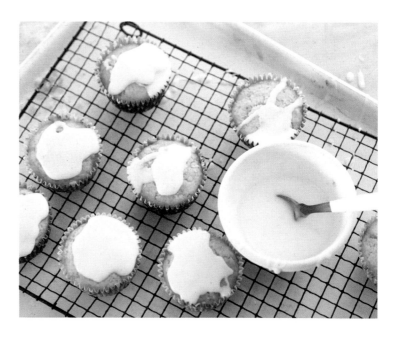

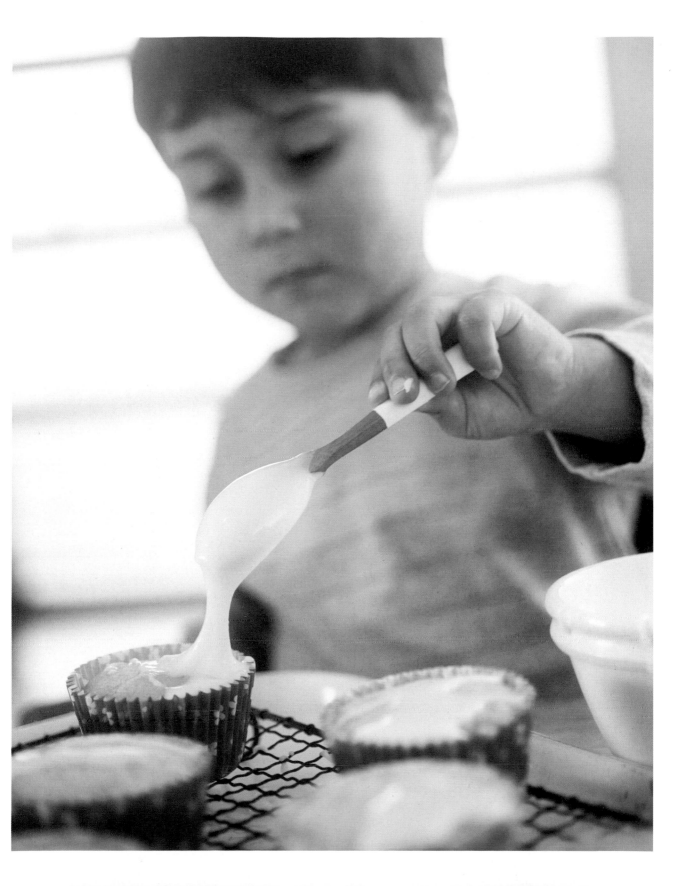

cherry crumble muffins

Makes 12

Preparation time 10 minutes

Cooking time 20 minutes

250 g (8 oz) brown rice flour

1 teaspoon bicarbonate of soda

2 teaspoons gluten-free baking powder

125 g (4 oz) golden caster sugar

300 g (10 oz) can black cherries, drained

75 g (3 oz) butter, melted

2 eggs, beaten

150 ml (¼ pint) buttermilk

Topping

1 tablespoon ground almonds

1 tablespoon soft light brown sugar

1 tablespoon brown rice flour

15 g (½ oz) butter

1 Line a 12-hole muffin tray with muffin cases.

2 Sift the flour, bicarbonate of soda and baking powder into a large bowl, then stir in the sugar. Mix together the cherries, melted butter, eggs and buttermilk in a separate bowl, then pour into the dry ingredients and stir gently until just combined. Spoon the mixture into the muffin cases.

3 Place the topping ingredients in a food processor and whizz until the mixture resembles fine breadcrumbs. Alternatively, mix together the ground almonds, sugar and flour in a bowl. Add the butter and rub in with the finegrtips until the mixture resembles fine breadcrumbs. Sprinkle over the muffin mixture.

4 Place in a preheated oven, 180°C (350°F), Gas Mark 4, for 20 minutes until golden and firm to the touch. Transfer to a wire rack to cool.

apricot & saffron muffins

Makes 12

Preparation time 10 minutes, plus cooling

Cooking time 25 minutes

100 g (3½ oz) ready-to-eat dried apricots,
  roughly chopped

grated rind and juice of 1 orange

pinch of saffron threads

300 g (10 oz) rice flour

2 teaspoons gluten-free baking powder

150 g (5 oz) golden caster sugar

125 ml (4 fl oz) sunflower oil

225 ml (7½ fl oz) buttermilk

2 large eggs, beaten

25 g (1 oz) flaked almonds

Topping

200 g (7 oz) cream cheese

2 tablespoons icing sugar

2 tablespoons clear honey

1 Line a 12-hole muffin tray with muffin cases.

2 Place the apricots, orange juice and rind and saffron in a small saucepan and simmer for 5 minutes until tender. Tip into a food processor or blender and whizz to a purée. Set aside.

3 Mix the flour, baking powder and sugar in a large bowl. Whisk together the oil, buttermilk and eggs then pour into the dry ingredients. Add the apricot purée and stir until just combined.

4 Spoon the mixture into the muffin cases and sprinkle with the almonds. Place in a preheated oven, 180°C (350°F), Gas Mark 4, for about 20 minutes until golden and springy to the touch. Transfer to a wire rack to cool.

5 Beat together the topping ingredients in a bowl, then spread over the cooled muffins.

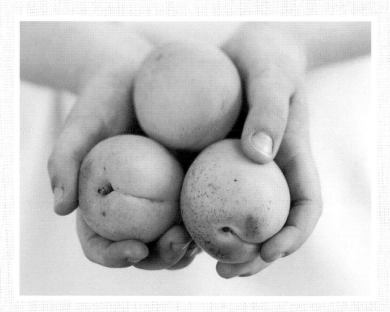

velvet cupcakes with marshmallow topping

Makes 12

Preparation time 20 minutes, plus cooling

Cooking time 25–30 minutes

200 g (7 oz) brown rice flour

2 tablespoons cornflour

3 tablespoons cocoa powder, sifted

2 teaspoons gluten-free baking powder

½ teaspoon bicarbonate of soda

75 g (3 oz) butter, softened

175 g (6 oz) caster sugar

2 heaped teaspoons red food colouring paste

few drops of vanilla extract

2 eggs, beaten

200 ml (7 fl oz) buttermilk

1 teaspoon white wine vinegar

crumbled, freeze-dried raspberries, to serve

Marshmallow icing

250 g (8 oz) caster sugar

4 tablespoons golden syrup

4 tablespoons water

4 large egg whites

1 Line a 12-hole muffin tray with cupcake cases.

2 Stir together the flours, cocoa powder, baking powder and bicarbonate of soda in a bowl.

3 Beat together the butter and sugar in a large bowl until pale and fluffy, then stir in the food colouring and vanilla extract. Gradually add the eggs, then stir in the buttermilk and vinegar. Fold in the flour mixture.

4 Spoon the mixture into the paper cases and place in a preheated oven, 180°C (350°F), Gas Mark 4, for 15–18 minutes until risen and just firm to the touch. Transfer to a wire rack to cool.

5 Make the marshmallow icing. Place the sugar, syrup and measurement water in a large saucepan and heat gently, stirring, until the sugar has dissolved. Bring to the boil and simmer for about 5 minutes until the mixture reaches 115°C (240°F). Remove the pan from the heat.

6 Whisk the egg whites in a large clean bowl until they form stiff peaks, then gradually pour in the syrup mixture, whisking continuously for 10 minutes until the icing is thick and glossy. Smooth icing over cooled cakes using the back of the spoon.

7 Sprinkle over the freeze-dried raspberries.

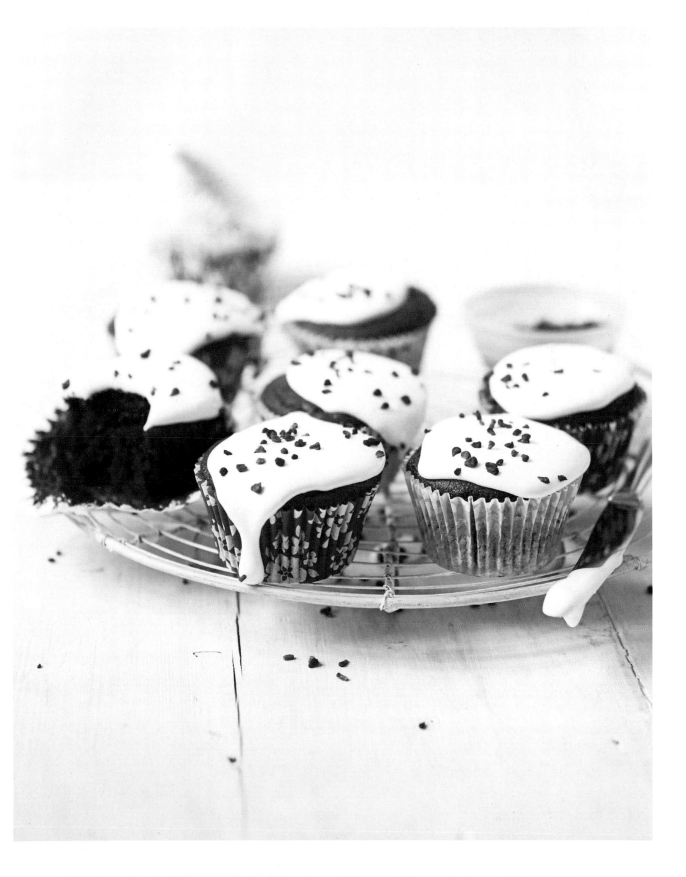

st clement's madeleines

Makes 12

Preparation time 10 minutes, plus standing

Cooking time 8–10 minutes

butter, for greasing

75 g (3 oz) rice flour, plus extra for dusting

2 eggs

75 g (3 oz) caster sugar

25 g (1 oz) cornflour

½ teaspoon gluten-free baking powder

grated rind of 1 lemon

grated rind of 1 orange

100 g (3½ oz) butter, melted

icing sugar, for dusting

These are best eaten warm soon after baking and are delicious with a glass of milk.

1 Grease and flour a 12-hole madeleine tin. Alternatively, grease and flour 20 holes of a mini muffin tin.

2 Whisk together the eggs and sugar in a large bowl until pale and creamy. Gently fold in all the remaining ingredients, then leave to stand for 20 minutes.

3 Spoon the mixture into the prepared tin and place in a preheated oven, 200°C (400°F), Gas Mark 6, for 8–10 minutes until springy to touch. Tip out on to a wire rack to cool slightly and lightly dust with icing sugar. Serve warm.

Tips and tricks

Try adding a tablespoon of cocoa powder to the mixture before resting to make chocolate orange madeleines.

orange & forest fruit friands

Makes 6

Preparation time 10 minutes

Cooking time 15–20 minutes

3 egg whites

125 g (4 oz) icing sugar, plus extra for dusting

25 g (1 oz) rice flour

100 g (3½ oz) ground almonds

100 g (3½ oz) butter, melted

grated rind of 1 orange

12 blackberries

24 raspberries

1 Line a 6-hole muffin tray or friand tin with paper cases. Alternatively, grease the tins with butter.

2 Whisk the egg whites in a large clean bowl until they are fluffy but not forming peaks. Stir in all the remaining ingredients except the fruit. Spoon the mixture into the paper cases and top with the fruit.

3 Place in a preheated oven, 180°C (350°F), Gas Mark 4, for about 15–20 minutes until golden and slightly springy to the touch.

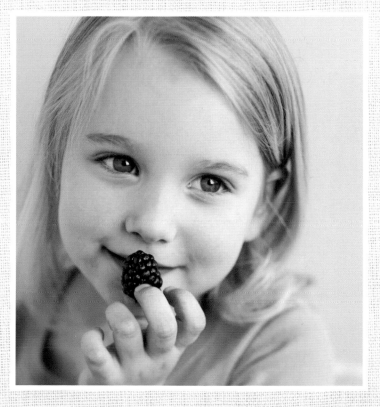

banana & peanut brownies

Makes 16

Preparation time 10 minutes

Cooking time 30–40 minutes

150 g (5 oz) butter, plus extra for greasing

200 g (7 oz) gluten-free plain dark chocolate, broken into pieces

175 g (6 oz) caster sugar

2 eggs

2 small ripe bananas, mashed

100 g (3½ oz) rice flour

1 teaspoon gluten-free baking powder

100 g (3½ oz) gluten-free white chocolate chips

3 tablespoons crunchy peanut butter

Icing sugar, for dusting

1 Grease and line a 20 cm (8 inch) square cake tin.

2 Melt the butter and dark chocolate in a large heatproof bowl set over a saucepan of gently simmering water, ensuring the bottom of the bowl does not touch the water.

3 Beat together the sugar and eggs in a separate large bowl until pale and fluffy, then stir in the bananas, flour, baking powder and chocolate chips. Fold in the melted chocolate mixture.

4 Pour the mixture into the prepared tin, then dot over the peanut butter and swirl with a knife. Place in a preheated oven, 180°C (350°F), Gas Mark 4, for 25–35 minutes until softly set. Leave to cool in the tin on a wire rack, then turn out and cut into squares. Serve dusted with icing sugar.

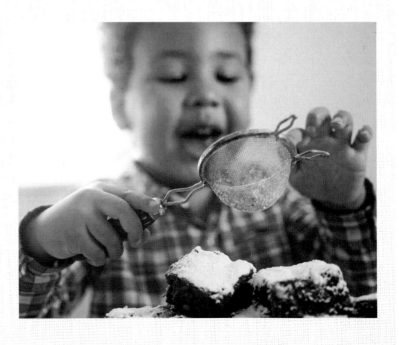

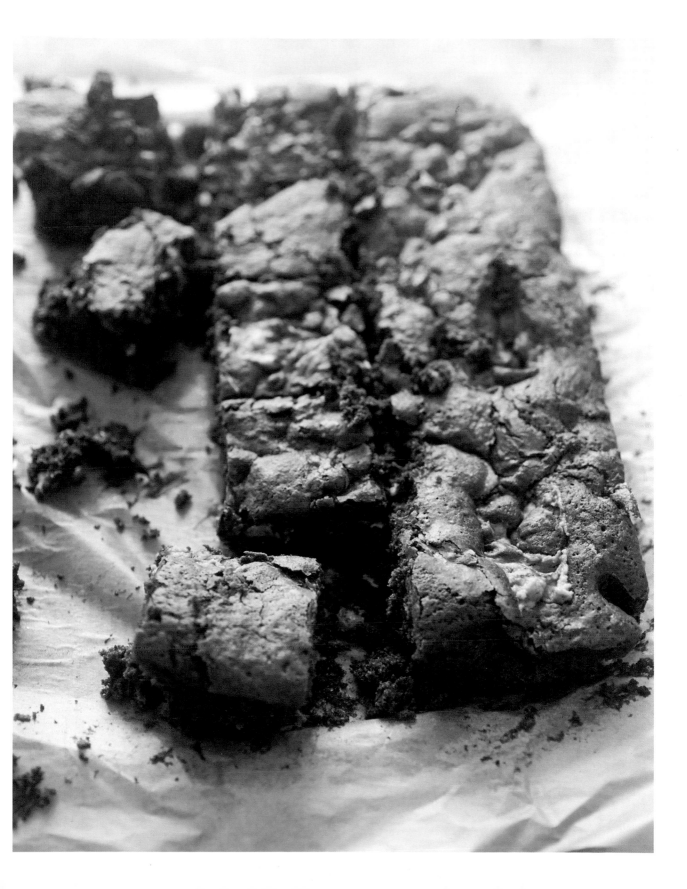

polenta cake with zesty curd & mascarpone topping

Serves 12

Preparation time 10 minutes, plus cooling

Cooking time 1–1¼ hours

250 g (8 oz) butter, softened, plus extra
 for greasing

200 g (7 oz) golden caster sugar

125 g (4 oz) fine polenta

1 teaspoon gluten-free baking powder

200 g (7 oz) ground almonds

3 eggs, beaten

grated rind 2 oranges

Topping

250 g (8 oz) mascarpone cheese

4 tablespoons Lemon, Orange & Passion
 Fruit Curd (*see* page 30) or gluten-free
 lemon curd

1 Lightly grease and line a 23 cm (9 inch) round deep cake tin.

2 Beat together the butter and sugar in a large bowl until pale and fluffy. Add all the remaining ingredients and combine until smooth.

3 Pour the mixture into the prepared tin and place in a preheated oven, 170°C (325°F), Gas Mark 3, for 1–1¼ hours until golden and a skewer inserted into the centre comes out clean. Transfer to a wire rack to cool.

4 Beat together the mascarpone and the fruit curd in a bowl, then spread over the cooled cake.

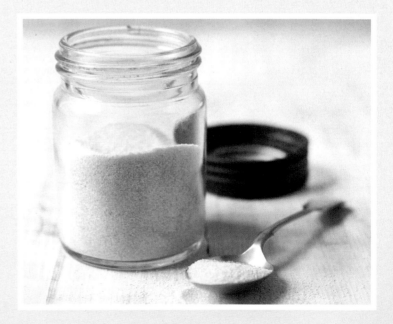

lemon drizzle loaf

Serves 12

Preparation time 15 minutes

Cooking time 35–40 minutes

250 g (8 oz) butter, softened, plus extra
  for greasing

250 g (8 oz) caster sugar

250 g (8 oz) brown rice flour

2 teaspoons gluten-free baking powder

4 eggs, beaten

grated rind and juice of 1 lemon

lemon rind twist, to decorate (optional)

Lemon drizzle

grated rind and juice of 2 lemons

100 g (3½ oz) granulated sugar

1 Grease and line a 900 g (2 lb) loaf tin.

2 Place all the cake ingredients except the lemon rind twist, if using, in a food processor and whizz until smooth or beat together in a large bowl.

3 Spoon the mixture into the prepared tin and place in a preheated oven, 180°C (350°F), Gas Mark 4, for 35–40 minutes until golden and firm to the touch.

4 Prick holes all over the sponge with a cocktail stick. Mix together the drizzle ingredients in a bowl, then drizzle the liquid over the warm loaf. Leave until completely cold. Decorate with a twist of lemon rind, if liked.

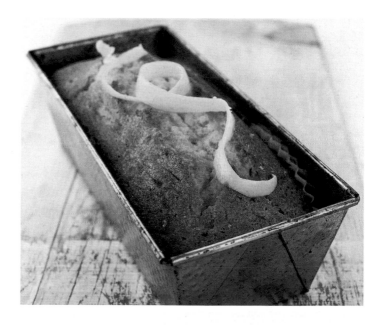

pear traybake

Serves 12

Preparation time 10 minutes

Cooking time 45 minutes

150 g (5 oz) butter, softened, plus extra
 for greasing

300 g (10 oz) brown rice flour

2 teaspoons gluten-free baking powder

1 teaspoon ground cinnamon

200 g (7 oz) soft light brown sugar

4 eggs

150 ml (¼ pint) buttermilk

3 pears, peeled, cored and sliced

Crumble topping

2 tablespoons brown rice flour

25 g (1 oz) cold butter, cubed

1 tablespoon demerara sugar

This will be just as popular with adults as it is with kids and is the perfect accompaniment to a cup of tea.

1 Grease and line a 20 x 30 cm (8 x 12 inch) baking tin.

2 Place all the sponge ingredients except the pears in a food processor and whizz until smooth or beat together in a large bowl. Pour the mixture into the prepared tin, then arrange the pears on top.

3 Make the crumble topping. Place the flour in a bowl, add the butter and rub in with the fingertips until the mixture resembles fine breadcrumbs. Stir in the sugar, then sprinkle it all over the top of the cake mixture.

4 Place in a preheated oven, 180°C (350°F), Gas Mark 4, for about 45 minutes until golden and just firm to the touch.

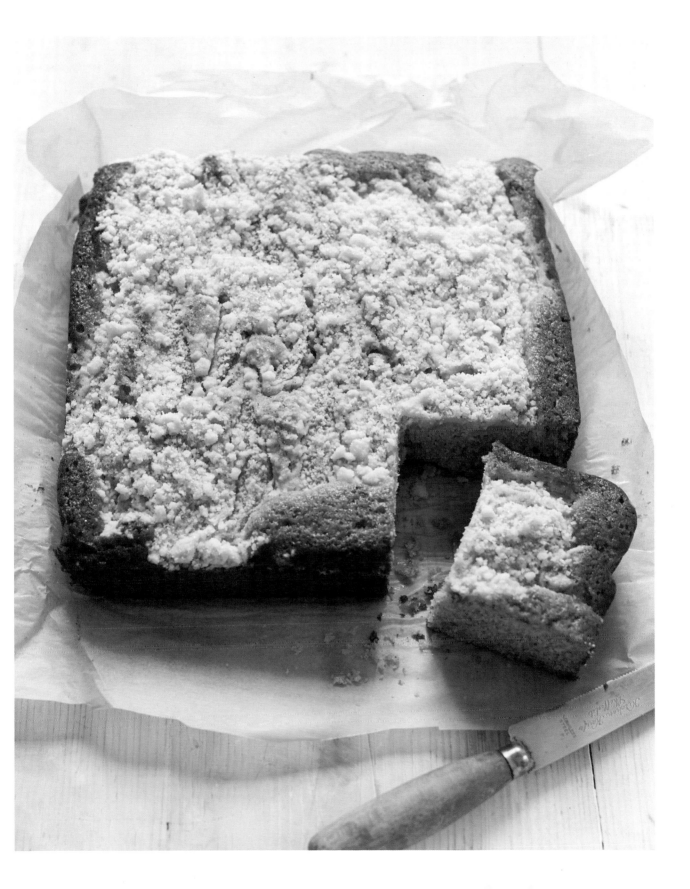

coconut & mango cake

Serves 12

Preparation time 15 minutes, plus cooling

Cooking time 45–50 minutes

100 g (3½ oz) butter, softened, plus extra
  for greasing

100 g (3½ oz) soft light brown sugar

4 eggs, separated

400 ml (14 fl oz) buttermilk

200 g (7 oz) polenta

200 g (7 oz) rice flour

2 teaspoons gluten-free baking powder

50 g (2 oz) coconut milk powder

50 g (2 oz) desiccated coconut

1 mango, peeled, stoned and puréed

Filling

250 g (8 oz) mascarpone cheese

1 mango, peeled, stoned and finely
  chopped

2 tablespoons icing sugar

1 Grease and line a 23 cm (9 inch) round deep cake tin.

2 Beat together the butter and sugar in a large bowl until pale and fluffy, then beat in the egg yolks, buttermilk, polenta, flour, baking powder, coconut milk powder and desiccated coconut.

3 Whisk the egg whites in a large clean bowl until they form soft peaks, then fold into the cake mixture with the puréed mango.

4 Spoon the mixture into the prepared tin and place in a preheated oven, 200°C (400°F), Gas Mark 6, for 45–50 minutes until golden and firm to the touch. Transfer to a wire rack to cool.

5 Slice the cooled cake in half horizontally. Beat together all the filling ingredients in a bowl and spread half over 1 sponge, then sandwich together with the remaining sponge. Spread the remaining mixture over the top.

victoria sandwich cake

Serves 12

Preparation time 10 minutes, plus cooling

Cooking time 20 minutes

175 g (6 oz) butter, softened, plus extra
for greasing

175 g (6 oz) caster sugar

175 g (6 oz) brown rice flour, plus extra
for dusting

3 eggs

1 tablespoon gluten-free baking powder

few drops of vanilla extract

1 tablespoon milk

To decorate

4 tablespoons raspberry jam

icing sugar

1 Grease and flour 2 x 18 cm (7 inch) round cake tins.

2 Place all the cake ingredients in a food processor and whizz
until smooth or beat together in a large bowl.

3 Spoon the mixture into the prepared tins and place in a
preheated oven, 200°C (400°F), Gas Mark 6, for about 20 minutes
until risen and golden. Transfer to a wire rack to cool.

4 Sandwich the cooled cakes together with the jam and dust
with icing sugar.

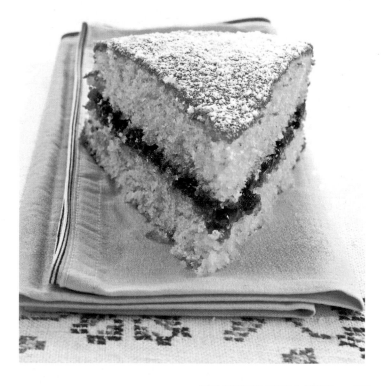

cranberry cookies

Makes 30

Preparation time 10 minutes

Cooking time 12–15 minutes

100 g (3½ oz) polyunsaturated margarine

100 g (3½ oz) soft light brown sugar

1 egg, beaten

125 g (4 oz) rice flour

100 g (3½ oz) buckwheat flour

50 g (2 oz) millet flakes

50 g (2 oz) dried cranberries, chopped dried apricots or raisins

For a treat, throw in some gluten-free chocolate chips with the fruit for fruity chocolate cookies.

1 Grease 3 baking sheets.

2 Beat together the margarine and sugar in a large bowl. Beat in the egg, then stir in all the remaining ingredients and combine to form a dough.

3 Place walnut-sized balls of the dough on a baking sheet and press down with a fork.

4 Place in a preheated oven, 180°C (350°F), Gas Mark 4, for 12–15 minutes until golden. Transfer to a wire rack to cool.

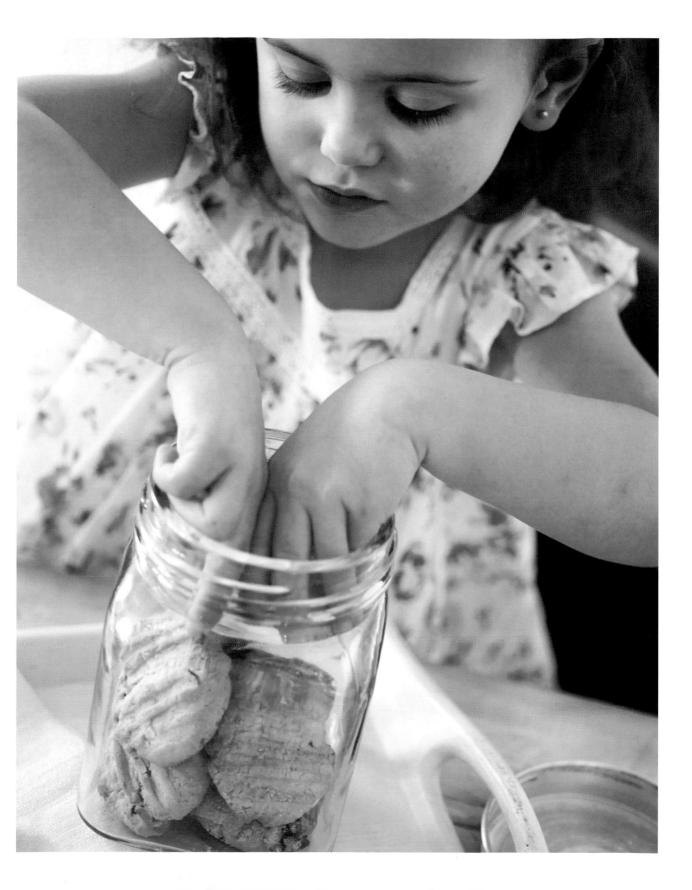

banana flapjacks

Makes 12

Preparation time 5–10 minutes

Cooking time 20–25 minutes

100 g (3½ oz) butter, melted, plus extra
for greasing

2 large ripe bananas

150 g (5 oz) dates, chopped

2 tablespoons golden syrup

200 g (7 oz) millet flakes

75 g (3 oz) hazelnuts, toasted and roughly
chopped

1 Lightly grease a 20 cm (8 inch) square baking tin.

2 Place the bananas in a bowl and mash well, then stir in all the remaining ingredients.

3 Press into the prepared tin and place in a preheated oven, 180°C (350°F), Gas Mark 4, for 20–25 minutes until golden.

4 Leave in the tin and mark into 12 bars, then leave to cool in the tin before turning out and breaking into bars.

Tips and tricks

These will work well with any nuts that you have to hand. You can also include dried cranberries for an extra berry boost.

chocolate chip cookies

Makes 30

Preparation time 10 minutes

Cooking time 8–10 minutes

75 g (3 oz) butter, softened, plus extra for greasing

100 g (3½ oz) caster sugar

75 g (3 oz) soft light brown sugar

1 egg, beaten

150 g (5 oz) brown rice flour, plus extra for dusting

½ teaspoon bicarbonate of soda

1 tablespoon cocoa powder

75 g (3 oz) gluten-free plain dark chocolate chips

1 Grease 3 baking sheets.

2 Put all the ingredients except the chocolate chips in a food processor and whizz until smooth or beat together in a large bowl. Stir in the chocolate chips, then bring the mixture together to form a ball.

3 Turn the dough out on a surface lightly dusted with rice flour and divide into 30 equal-sized balls. Place on the prepared sheets, well spaced apart, pressing down gently with the back of a fork.

4 Place in a preheated oven, 180°C (350°F), Gas Mark 4, for 8–10 minutes. Leave to harden on the baking sheets for a few minutes, then transfer to a wire rack to cool.

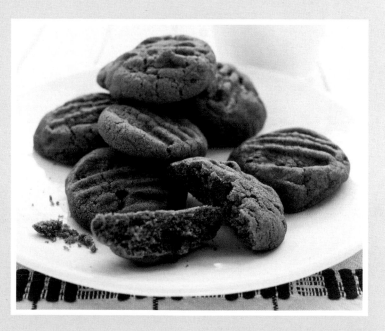

buttery shortbread

Makes 12

Preparation time 10 minutes

Cooking time 10–12 minutes

100 g (3½ oz) butter, softened, plus extra
   for greasing

50 g (2 oz) golden caster sugar

100 g (3½ oz) rice flour

100 g (3½ oz) cornflour

demerara sugar, for sprinkling

1 Grease a 28 x 18 cm (11 x 7 inch) baking tin.

2 Beat together the butter and sugar in a bowl until pale and fluffy, then stir in the flours and combine to form a dough.

3 Press the dough into the prepared tin and prick all over with a fork. Sprinkle over the demerara sugar.

4 Place in a preheated oven, 200°C (400°F), Gas Mark 6, for 10–12 minutes until golden.

5 Leave in the tin and mark into 12 bars, then leave to cool in the tin before turning out and breaking into bars.

Tips and tricks

This basic shortbread recipe can be varied. Try chocolate shortbread – replace the rice and cornflour with buckwheat flour and add 2 tablespoons cocoa powder. Or you could make nutty spiced shortbread – add 1 teaspoon mixed spice and the grated rind of 1 orange to the basic mixture, then press 150 g (5 oz) chopped mixed nuts into the dough after it has been pressed into the tin.

fruity mango flapjacks

Makes 12

Preparation time 10 minutes

Cooking time 35 minutes

150 g (5 oz) butter, plus extra for greasing

100 g (3½ oz) soft light brown sugar

2 tablespoons golden syrup

200 g (7 oz) millet flakes

2 tablespoons mixed pumpkin and sunflower seeds

75 g (3 oz) dried mango, roughly chopped

1 Grease a 28 x 18 cm (11 x 7 inch) baking tin.

2 Place the sugar, butter and syrup in a heavy-based saucepan and heat until melted, then stir in the remaining ingredients.

3 Spoon the mixture into the prepared tin and press down lightly. Place in a preheated oven, 150°C (300°F), Gas Mark 2, for 30 minutes.

4 Leave in the tin and mark into 12 bars, then place on a wire rack to cool completely before turning out and breaking into bars.

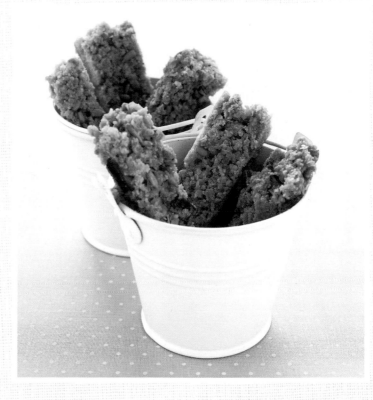

basic white loaf

Makes 1 loaf

Preparation time 10 minutes, plus proving

Cooking time 35–40 minutes

1 x 7g (¼ oz) sachet fast-action dried yeast

1 tablespoon caster sugar

300 ml (½ pint) warm water

½ teaspoon salt

1 teaspoon gluten-free baking powder

4 tablespoons dried milk powder

150 g (5 oz) potato starch

300 g (10 oz) rice flour

6 tablespoons cornflour

1 tablespoon xanthan gum

2 eggs, beaten

4 tablespoons vegetable oil

1 Line a 900 g (2 lb) loaf tin.

2 Put the yeast, sugar and 100 ml (3½ fl oz) of the warm water in a jug and set aside for about 10 minutes until frothy.

3 Stir together the salt, baking powder, milk powder, potato starch, flours and xanthan gum in a large bowl. Mix together the eggs, oil and remaining water in a separate bowl, then stir into the yeast mixture and add to the dry ingredients. Combine to form a dough, adding a little extra water or flour if necessary.

4 Pour into the prepared tin and level the top. Spritz with a little water, then leave in a warm place to rise for about 1½ hours until it comes to the top of the tin.

5 Place in a preheated oven, 200°C (400°F), Gas Mark 6, for 15 minutes, then reduce the temperature to 180°C (350°F), Gas Mark 4 and bake for a further 20–25 minutes until the loaf is golden and firm to touch. Leave to cool in the tin for 10 minutes, then tip out on to a wire rack to cool.

cheese, apple & walnut bread

Makes 1 loaf

Preparation time 15 minutes

Cooking time 40–45 minutes

250 g (8 oz) rice flour, plus extra for dusting

200 g (7 oz) buckwheat flour

40 g (1½ oz) cold butter, cubed

1 large dessert apple, peeled, cored and finely chopped

150 g (5 oz) mature Cheddar cheese, grated

75 g (3 oz) walnuts, roughly chopped

2 tablespoons chopped chives

8–10 tablespoons skimmed milk

beaten egg, to glaze

salt and black pepper

1 Lightly dust a baking sheet with rice flour.

2 Sift the flours into a large bowl, tipping any bran remaining in the sieve into the bowl. Add the butter and rub in with the fingertips until the mixture resembles fine breadcrumbs. Season well. Using a fork, stir in the apple, cheese, walnuts and chives, then add enough of the milk to form a soft dough.

3 Turn the dough out on a surface lightly dusted with rice flour and shape into a round about 20 cm (8 inches) in diameter. Brush with the beaten egg, then cut a lattice pattern into the top using a sharp knife.

4 Transfer to the prepared baking sheet and place in a preheated oven, 190°C (375°F), Gas Mark 5, for 35–40 minutes until golden. Turn the loaf over and bake for a further 5 minutes. Serve warm.

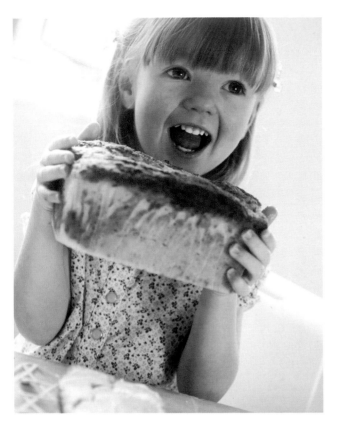
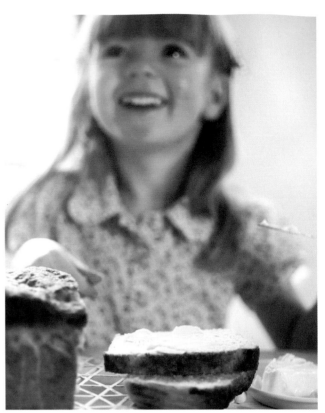
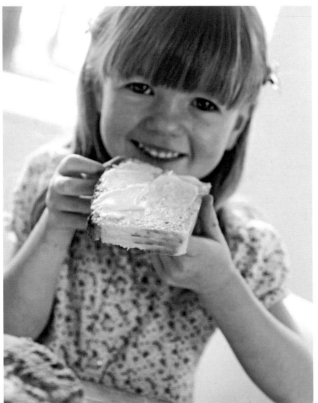
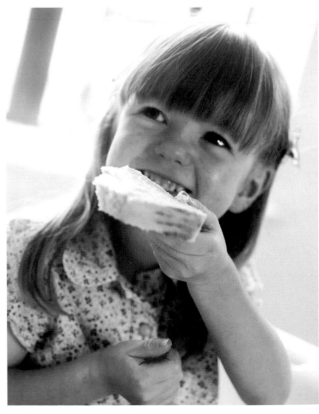

cheesy bread

Makes 1 loaf

Preparation time 10 minutes, plus proving

Cooking time 45 minutes

200 g (7 oz) polenta

100 g (3½ oz) rice flour

50 g (2 oz) dried milk powder

7 g (¼ oz) sachet fast-action dried yeast

1 teaspoon caster sugar

2 teaspoons xanthan gum

4 tablespoons grated Parmesan cheese

100 g (3½ oz) mature Cheddar cheese, grated

3 eggs, beaten

450 ml (¾ pint) hand-hot water

1 Line a 900 g (2 lb) loaf tin.

2 Stir together the polenta, flour, milk powder, yeast, sugar, xanthan gum and cheeses in a large bowl. Mix together the eggs and water in a jug, then pour into the dry ingredients and stir together to form a sticky dough.

3 Pour the mixture into the prepared tin, cover with a clean damp tea towel and leave to rise in a warm place for 30–45 minutes until the mixture is near the top of the tin.

4 Place in a preheated oven, 180°C (350°F), Gas Mark 4, for about 45 minutes or until golden and it sounds hollow when tapped on the base. Transfer to a wire rack to cool.

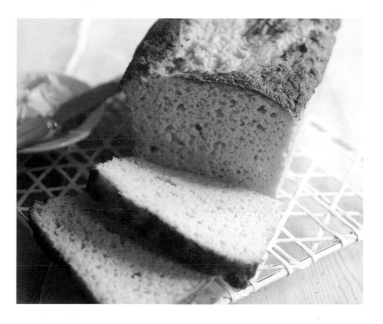

cheesy herby muffins

Makes 8

Preparation time 10 minutes

Cooking time 20 minutes

175 g (6 oz) Gruyère cheese, grated

3 spring onions, finely sliced

1 teaspoon thyme leaves

1 tablespoon chopped parsley

100 g (3½ oz) rice flour

½ teaspoon gluten-free baking powder

150 g (5 oz) fresh gluten-free
   breadcrumbs

1 teaspoon gluten-free English mustard

3 eggs, beaten

50 g (2 oz) butter, melted

4 tablespoons milk

1 Line 8 holes of a muffin tray with muffin cases.

2 Mix together all the ingredients in a large bowl until just combined.

3 Spoon the mixture into the muffin cases and place in a preheated oven, 190°C (375°F), Gas Mark 5, for 20 minutes or until golden and just firm to the touch. Serve warm.

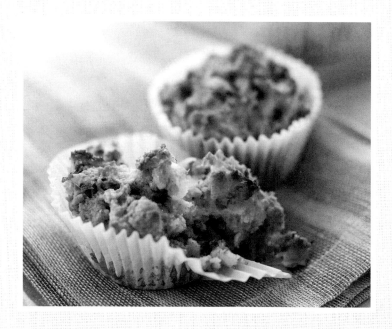

corn & bacon muffins

Makes 12

Preparation time 10 minutes

Cooking time 20–25 minutes

3 tablespoons vegetable oil, plus extra for greasing

6 streaky bacon rashers, finely chopped

1 small red onion, finely chopped

200 g (7 oz) frozen sweetcorn

175 g (6 oz) fine cornmeal

125 g (4 oz) rice flour

2 teaspoons gluten-free baking powder

50 g (2 oz) Cheddar cheese, grated

200 ml (7 fl oz) milk

2 eggs, beaten

1 Grease a 12-hole muffin tray with oil.

2 Heat a frying pan, add the bacon and onion and dry-fry for 3–4 minutes until the bacon is turning crisp.

3 Meanwhile, cook the sweetcorn in a saucepan of boiling water for 2 minutes to soften. Drain well.

4 Mix together the cornmeal, flour and baking powder in a bowl, then stir in the sweetcorn, cheese, bacon and onion. Whisk together the milk, eggs and oil in a jug, then pour into the dry ingredients and stir until just combined.

5 Pour the mixture into the holes in the prepared tray and place in a preheated oven, 220°C (425°F), Gas Mark 7, for 15–20 minutes until golden and just firm to the touch. Transfer to a wire rack to cool.

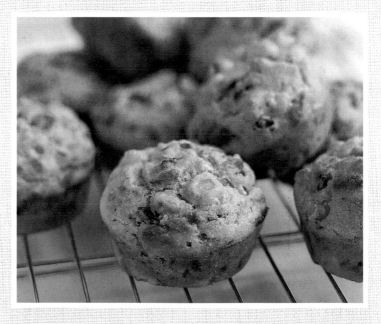

soda bread

Makes 1 loaf

Preparation time 10 minutes

Cooking time 30–35 minutes

250 g (8 oz) white rice flour, plus extra for dusting

100 g (3½ oz) tapioca flour

1 tablespoon caster sugar

2 tablespoons dried milk powder

1 teaspoon bicarbonate of soda

1 teaspoon gluten-free baking powder

1 teaspoon salt

1 egg, beaten

284 ml (10 fl oz) buttermilk

This loaf is so easy to make and lovely served hot with butter or toasted, perfect for Sunday afternoon tea.

1 Sift all the dry ingredients into a large bowl. Whisk together the egg and buttermilk in a jug, then stir into the dry ingredients and use your fingertips to form a dough.

2 Turn the dough out on a surface lightly dusted with rice flour and shape into a round. Place on a dusted baking sheet and make a large cross across the top of the dough using a sharp knife. Sprinkle over a little extra flour.

3 Place in an oven preheated to its highest setting for 5 minutes. Reduce the temperature to 180°C (350°F), Gas Mark 4, and bake for a further 25–30 minutes or until it sounds hollow when tapped on the base.

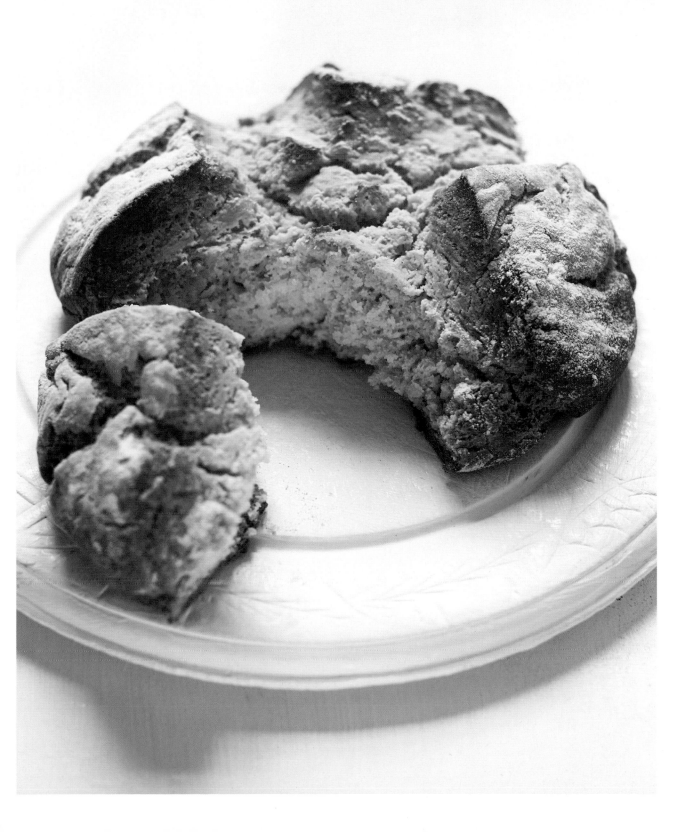

simple banoffee cheesecake

Serves 4

Preparation time 10 minutes, plus chilling

150 g (5 oz) amaretti biscuits, or other gluten-free biscuits, crushed

50 g (2 oz) butter, melted

3 bananas, sliced

280 g (10 oz) cream cheese

2 tablespoons icing sugar

6 tablespoons dulce de leche or canned caramel

This combination of two favourite desserts is delicious and indulgent, a real winner for all the family.

1 Mix together the crushed biscuits and melted butter in a bowl, then press into a 20 cm (8 inch) loose-bottomed or spring-form tin. Chill for 20 minutes.

2 Arrange the sliced bananas over the biscuit base. Beat together all the remaining ingredients in a bowl, then spread over the bananas.

3 Chill for at least 30 minutes before serving.

spiced pear & apple crumble

Serves 4

Preparation time 10 minutes

Cooking time 30–35 minutes

750 g (1½ lb) pears, peeled, cored and
  sliced

500 g (1 lb) cooking apples, peeled, cored
  and sliced

2 tablespoons soft light brown sugar

1 teaspoon ground cinnamon

4 tablespoons apple juice

crème fraîche or cream, to serve

Topping

200 g (7 oz) rice flour

100 g (3½ oz) cold butter, cubed

100 g (3½ oz) soft light brown sugar

25 g (1oz) flaked almonds

25 g (1 oz) blanched hazelnuts, roughly
  chopped

1 Put the pears and apples in a large saucepan with the sugar, cinnamon and apple juice. Cover and cook gently for about 10 minutes, stirring occasionally, until the fruit is just tender. Transfer to an ovenproof dish.

2 Make the topping. Place the flour and butter in a food processor and whizz until the mixture resembles fine breadcrumbs. Alternatively, place the flour in a large bowl, add the butter and rub in with the fingertips until the mixture resembles fine breadcrumbs. Stir in the sugar and nuts, then sprinkle over the fruit and press down gently.

3 Place in a preheated oven, 200°C (400°F), Gas Mark 6, for 20–25 minutes until golden and bubbling. Serve with crème fraîche or cream.

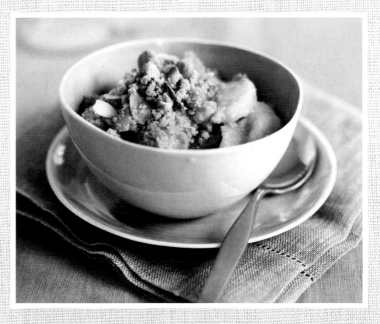

rhubarb & custard ice cream

Serves 6

Preparation time 15 minutes, plus cooling and freezing

Cooking time 20 minutes

450 g (14½ oz) rhubarb, cut into 5 cm (2½ inch) chunks

300 g (10 oz) caster sugar

2 tablespoons water

5 egg yolks

300 ml (½ pint) double cream

300 ml (½ pint) milk

few drops of vanilla extract

1 Place the rhubarb, 75 g (3 oz) of the sugar and the measurement water in a small saucepan. Cover and cook over a low heat for about 10 minutes until the rhubarb is tender. Leave to cool slightly, then tip into a food processor or blender and blend to a purée. Set aside.

2 Whisk the remaining sugar and egg yolks in a heatproof bowl until thick and pale. Heat the cream, milk and vanilla extract in a saucepan until hot, then whisk into the sugar mixture. Return the mixture to the pan and heat gently, stirring continuously, until the custard is thickened – do not allow to boil.

3 Remove the pan from the heat, cover with clingfilm and leave the custard to cool.

4 When the custard is completely cold, stir in the rhubarb purée and tip into a freezerproof container. Freeze for 2 hours, then whisk the mixture to remove any ice crystals and return to the freezer for a further 2 hours. Whisk again, then freeze until solid.

rhubarb traybake

Serves 8

Preparation time 10 minutes

Cooking time 20 minutes

50 g (2 oz) polyunsaturated margarine, plus extra for greasing

2 tablespoons golden syrup

1 tablespoon soft light brown sugar

75 g (3 oz) millet flakes

50 g (2 oz) buckwheat flour

pinch of ground ginger

25 g (1 oz) pecan nuts, chopped

6 tablespoons rhubarb compote or stewed rhubarb (*see* Step 1 opposite)

1 Place the margarine, syrup and sugar in a saucepan and heat gently until the sugar has dissolved. Stir in the millet flakes, flour, ginger and pecans and combine well.

2 Press two-thirds of the mixture into a 15 cm (6 inch) square greased baking tin and gently press down. Spoon over the rhubarb, then sprinkle over the remaining millet mixture and press down lightly.

3 Place in a preheated oven, 180°C (350°F), Gas Mark 4, for 15–20 minutes until golden.

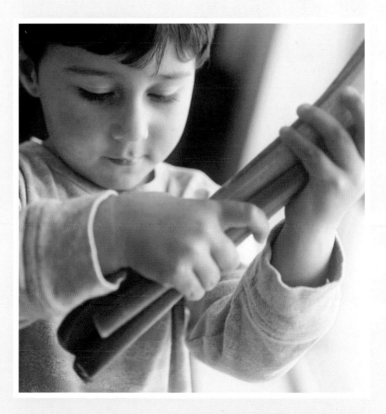

banana tarte tatin

Serves 6

Preparation time 15 minutes, plus chilling

Cooking time 30–35 minutes

50 g (2 oz) butter

100 g (3½ oz) caster sugar

5 firm bananas, halved lengthways

cream or ice cream, to serve

Pastry

125 g (4½ oz) rice flour, plus extra for
   dusting

2 tablespoons polenta

60 g (2¾ oz) cold butter, cubed

1 tablespoon caster sugar

1 egg yolk

1 Make the pastry. Place the flour, polenta, butter and sugar in a food processor and whizz until the mixture resembles fine breadcrumbs. Alternatively, mix together the rice flour and polenta in a large bowl. Add the butter and rub in with the fingertips until the mixture resembles fine breadcrumbs, then stir in the sugar. Add the egg yolk and enough water to form a dough.

2 Meanwhile, melt the butter in a heavy-based 22 cm (9 inch) ovenproof frying pan. Add the sugar and cook over a medium heat until it has turned a golden caramel colour. Leave to cool slightly, then arrange the bananas in the pan, cut side up (you may have to cut a few pieces a little smaller to fit the pan).

3 Turn the pastry out on a surface lightly dusted with rice flour and roll out to a round a little bigger than the tin. Lay the pastry over the bananas and tuck in the sides.

4 Place in a preheated oven, 220°C (425°F), Gas Mark 7, for 25–30 minutes or until golden and starting to bubble around the sides.

5 Carefully invert on to a serving plate and serve with cream or ice cream.

crunchy plum slump

Serves 4–6

Preparation time 15 minutes

Cooking time 20–25 minutes

650 g (1lb 7 oz) plums, halved, stoned and quartered

½ teaspoon ground ginger

50 g (2 oz) golden caster sugar

grated rind and juice of 1 orange

4 tablespoons mascarpone cheese

175 g (6 oz) brown rice flour

50 g (2 oz) butter or margarine, cubed

2 tablespoons light soft brown sugar

grated rind of ½ lemon

6 tablespoons milk

1 Place the plums, ginger, caster sugar and the orange rind and juice into a medium saucepan and bring to the boil, then simmer gently for 5–6 minutes until the plums are just tender. Tip into an ovenproof dish and spoon over blobs of mascarpone.

2 Place the flour in a bowl, add the butter or margarine and rub in with fingertips until the mixture resembles breadcrumbs. Stir in the brown sugar, lemon rind and milk until combined. Drop spoonfuls of the mixture over the plums and mascarpone.

3 Place in a preheated oven, 200°C (400°F), Gas Mark 6, for 15–20 minutes until golden and bubbling.

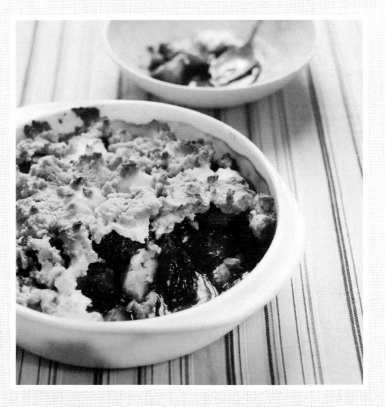

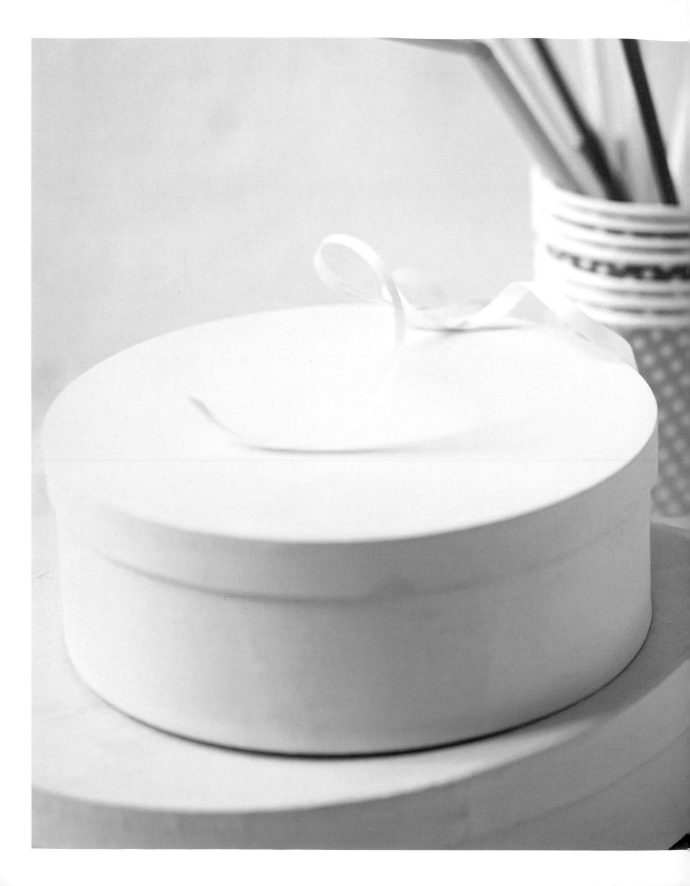

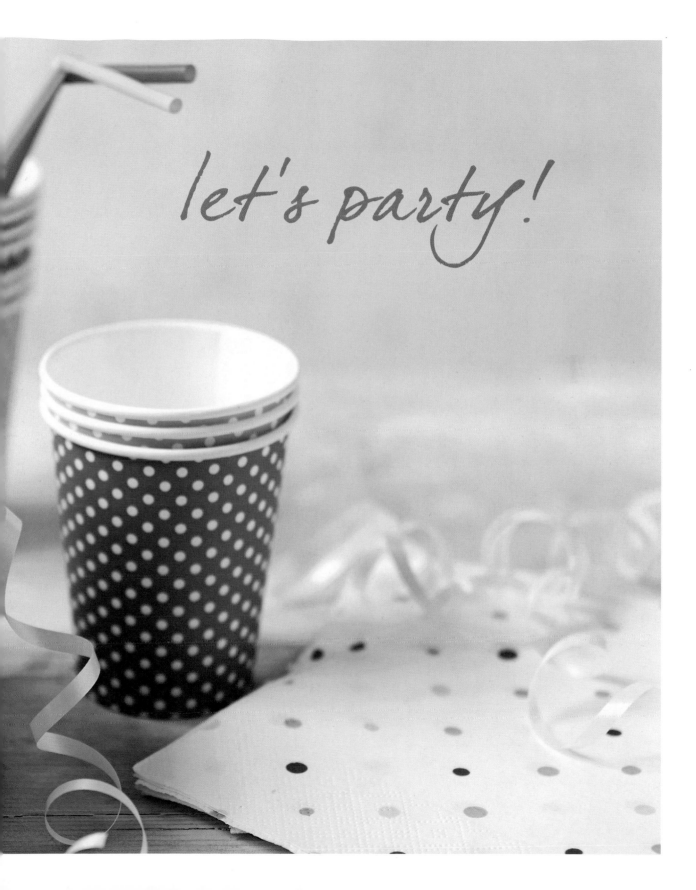

cheesy bites

Makes about 48

Preparation time 15 minutes, plus chilling

Cooking time 12–15 minutes

125 g (4 oz) rice flour, plus extra for
  dusting

50 g (2 oz) cornflour

100 g (3½ oz) cold butter, cubed

75 g (3 oz) mature Cheddar cheese, grated

2 tablespoons grated Parmesan cheese

1 egg yolk

1 Place the flours and butter in a food processor and whizz until the mixture resembles fine breadcrumbs. Alternatively, place the flours in a large bowl, add the butter and rub in with the fingertips until the mixture resembles fine breadcrumbs. Stir in the Cheddar and half of the Parmesan. Add the egg yolk and enough water to form a dough.

2 Turn the dough out on a surface lightly dusted with rice flour and roll out to a rectangle about 0.5 cm (¼ inch) thick. Cut out small shapes, such as stars or rounds (as these are very crumbly it is best to keep the shapes small so that the bites are more stable). Transfer to a greased baking sheet and sprinkle over the remaining Parmesan.

3 Place in a preheated oven, 180°C (350°F), Gas Mark 4, for 12–15 minutes until golden. Transfer to a wire rack to cool.

parmesan & mixed seed lollies

Makes 12

Preparation time 10 minutes

Cooking time 3–5 minutes

200 g (7 oz) Parmesan cheese, grated

2 tablespoons sesame seeds

1 tablespoon poppy seeds

1 tablespoon sunflower or pumpkin seeds

pinch of cayenne pepper (optional)

1 Line 2 baking sheets with nonstick baking paper.

2 Mix together all the ingredients in a bowl, then spoon on to the prepared baking sheets to form 12 piles, spaced well apart. Press a lolly stick into each pile so that part of the sticks are covered with a little of the mixture.

3 Place in a preheated oven, 200°C (400°F), Gas Mark 6, for 3–5 minutes until golden and lacy. Leave to cool on the baking sheets, then serve.

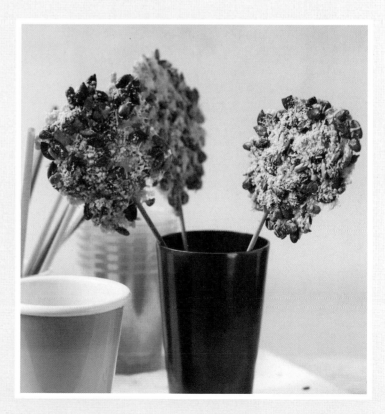

pizza scrolls

Makes 8

Preparation time 25 minutes, plus proving

Cooking time 12–15 minutes

2 x 7 g (¼ oz) sachets fast-action dried yeast

1 teaspoon caster sugar

250 ml (8 fl oz) milk, warmed

175 g (6 oz) rice flour, plus extra for dusting

125 g (4 oz) potato flour

1 teaspoon gluten-free baking powder

1 teaspoon xanthan gum

pinch of salt

1 tablespoon sunflower oil, plus extra for oiling

1 egg, beaten

Filling

4 tablespoons passata

200 g (7 oz) mixed mozzarella and Cheddar cheese, grated

75 g (3 oz) wafer-thin ham, shredded

handful of basil, chopped

1 Put the yeast, sugar and milk in a bowl and set aside for about 10 minutes until frothy.

2 Stir together the flours, baking powder, xanthan gum and salt in a large bowl. Mix together the oil and egg in a separate bowl, stir into the yeast mixture and add this to the dry ingredients. Combine to form a soft dough.

3 Turn the dough out on a surface lightly dusted with rice flour and knead for 5 minutes, adding a little rice flour if the mixture becomes sticky. Place in a lightly oiled bowl, cover with a clean damp tea towel and leave in a warm place to rise for 40 minutes or until well risen.

4 Lightly oil a heavy baking sheet or tin. Roll the dough out on the floured surface to a rectangle about 30 x 25 cm (12 x 10 inches), spread with the passata, then sprinkle over the remaining filling ingredients. Roll the pizza up from one long edge, then slice into 8 pieces.

5 Place the rolled-up pizza scrolls side by side on the prepared baking sheet or tin. They should be pushed up against each other so that the sides are touching. Place in a preheated oven, 220°C (425°F), Gas Mark 7, for 12–15 minutes until golden. Serve warm.

scrumptious sausage rolls

Makes 20

Preparation time 20 minutes, plus chilling

Cooking time 18–20 minutes

6 gluten-free sausages, skins removed

handful of fresh herbs, such as chives and parsley, chopped (optional)

milk, for brushing

Pastry

200 g (7 oz) brown rice flour, plus extra for dusting

50 g (2 oz) polenta

½ teaspoon xanthan gum

100 g (3½ oz) cold butter, cubed

1 egg yolk

1 Make the pastry. Place the flour, polenta, xanthan gum and butter in a food processor and whizz until the mixture resembles breadcrumbs. Alternatively, mix together the dry ingredients in a large bowl. Add the butter and rub in with the fingertips until the mixture resembles breadcrumbs. Add the egg yolk and enough water to form a dough. Knead the dough for a few minutes, then wrap in clingfilm and chill for 30 minutes.

2 Meanwhile, place the sausagemeat and herbs in a bowl and mix well.

3 Turn the pastry out on a surface lightly dusted with rice flour and roll out to a square about 24 x 48 cm (9½ x 18¾ inches). Cut in half to form 2 rectangles.

4 Divide the sausagemeat into 2 pieces and shape into long rolls the same length as the pastry. Lay 1 sausagemeat roll on each piece of pastry, then wet the pastry edges with milk and fold over and press down to encase the meat and seal the edges. Cut each strip into about 10 sausage rolls, then snip the top of each with scissors to make a V shape. Brush the sausage rolls with milk.

5 Transfer the sausage rolls to a greased baking sheet and place in a preheated oven, 200°C (400°F), Gas Mark 6, for 18–20 minutes until golden and cooked through.

mince pies kiddie style

Makes 12

Preparation time 15 minutes, plus chilling

Cooking time 15–20 minutes

100 g (3½ oz) sultanas

50 g (2 oz) dried mango, chopped

75 g (3 oz) almonds, toasted and chopped

2 tablespoons clear honey

2 tablespoons cream cheese

milk, for brushing

Pastry

150 g (5 oz) rice flour, plus extra for
   dusting

25 g (1 oz) polenta

75 g (3 oz) cold butter, cubed

2 tablespoons caster sugar

1 egg yolk

grated rind of 1 orange

1 Make the pastry. Place the flour, polenta, butter and sugar in a food processor and whizz until the mixture resembles fine breadcrumbs. Alternatively, mix together the rice flour and polenta in a bowl. Add the butter and rub in with the fingertips until the mixture resembles fine breadcrumbs, then stir in the sugar. Add the egg, orange rind and enough cold water to form a dough. Wrap in clingfilm and chill for 30 minutes.

2 Mix together the sultanas, mango, almonds, honey and cream cheese in a bowl.

3 Roll the pastry out between 2 sheets of greaseproof paper or clingfilm. Cut out 12 rounds using a 7.5 cm (3 inch) pastry cutter and 12 rounds using a 6.5 cm (2½ inch) pastry cutter, rerolling the trimmings if necessary.

4 Use the large rounds to line a 12-hole bun tin. Divide the cream cheese mixture evenly among the cases, cover with the smaller pastry lids and press gently to seal the edges. Brush the tops with a little milk and cut a slit in each.

5 Place in a preheated oven, 180°C (350°F), Gas Mark 4, for 15–20 minutes until golden.

lemon & raspberry cupcakes

Makes 12

Preparation time 10 minutes

Cooking time 12–15 minutes

150 g (5 oz) butter, softened

150 g (5 oz) caster sugar

75 g (3 oz) rice flour

75 g (3 oz) cornflour

1 tablespoon gluten-free baking powder

grated rind and juice of 1 lemon

3 eggs, beaten

125 g (4 oz) raspberries

1 tablespoon gluten-free lemon curd

1 Line a 12-hole muffin tray with cupcake cases.

2 Whisk together all the ingredients except the raspberries and lemon curd in a large bowl. Fold in the raspberries.

3 Spoon half the sponge mixture into the muffin cases, dot over a little of the lemon curd, then share the remaining sponge mixture across the muffin cases.

4 Place in a preheated oven, 200°C (400°F), Gas Mark 6, for 12–15 minutes until golden and firm to the touch. Transfer to a wire rack to cool.

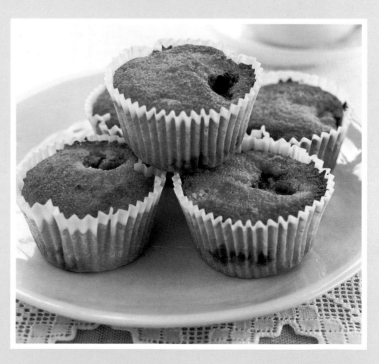

orange animal biscuits

Makes 20

Preparation time 15 minutes, plus cooling

Cooking time 10 minutes

200 g (7 oz) brown rice flour, plus extra for dusting

½ teaspoon xanthan gum

1 teaspoon gluten-free baking powder

50 g (2 oz) butter, cubed

50 g (2 oz) soft light brown sugar

grated rind of 1 orange

1 egg, beaten

2 tablespoons golden syrup

To decorate

150 g (5 oz) icing sugar

1 tablespoon boiling water

food colouring (optional)

gluten-free sweets

1 Line 2 baking sheets with nonstick baking paper.

2 Place the flour, xanthan gum, baking powder and butter in a food processor and whizz until the mixture resembles fine breadcrumbs. Alternatively, mix together the flour, xanthan gum and baking powder in a large bowl. Add the butter and rub in with the fingertips until the mixture resembles fine breadcrumbs. Stir in the sugar and orange rind. Add the egg and golden syrup and combine to form a firm dough.

3 Turn the dough out on a surface lightly dusted with rice flour and roll out to 5 mm (¼ inch) thick. Using animal cutters, cut out 20 biscuits, rerolling the trimmings as necessary.

4 Transfer the biscuits to the prepared baking sheets and place in a preheated oven, 160°C (325°F), Gas Mark 3, for about 10 minutes until golden. Leave to harden on the baking sheets for a few minutes, then transfer to a wire rack to cool.

5 Mix the icing sugar with the boiling water and add the colouring, if using, then smooth over the cooled biscuits or pipe icing details. Decorate with sweets and leave to set.

scary halloween cookies

Makes 12–14

Preparation time 15 minutes, plus cooling

Cooking time 12–15 minutes

100 g (3½ oz) butter, softened

100 g (3½ oz) soft light brown sugar

1 egg yolk

1 teaspoon ground ginger

200 g (7 oz) rice flour, plus extra for dusting

75 g (3 oz) cornflour

To decorate

300 g (10 oz) ready-to-roll icing

icing sugar, for dusting

icing pens

Use any shaped cookie cutter you like, such as bats or gingerbread men (you can cut off the heads, legs or arms to make them scarier). Choose icing colours to correspond with the cookie shapes – for example, black for bats.

1 Beat together the butter and sugar in a large bowl until pale and fluffy, then gradually beat in the egg yolk. Sift the ginger and flours into a separate bowl, then fold into the creamed mixture and form into a ball.

2 Turn the dough out on to a surface lightly dusted with rice flour and roll out to 5 mm (¼ inch) thick. Cut out shapes using cookie cutters, rerolling the trimmings if necessary, and transfer onto two baking sheets.

3 Place in a preheated oven, 190°C (375°F), Gas Mark 5, for 12–15 minutes until beginning to turn golden. Transfer to a wire rack to cool.

4 To decorate the cooled cookies, roll out the icing on a surface dusted with icing sugar and cut out shapes using the cookie cutters. Place on top of the cookies and add details using the icing pens.

chocolate sponge with buttercream

Serves 8

Preparation time 10 minutes, plus cooling

Cooking time 12–15 minutes

225 g (7½ oz) butter, softened, plus extra
  for greasing

225 g (7½ oz) caster sugar

200 g (7 oz) rice flour

25 g (1 oz) cocoa powder

4 eggs

2 teaspoons gluten-free baking powder

2 tablespoons milk

Icing

150 g (5 oz) butter, softened

250 g (8 oz) icing sugar

2 tablespoons cocoa powder

For a special occasion, decorate the cake with gluten-free sweets or crumbled flaky chocolate. If you prefer a vanilla sponge, increase the amount of rice flour by 25 g (1 oz) and replace the cocoa powder with a few drops of vanilla extract.

1 Lightly grease and line 2 x 20 cm (8 inch) sandwich tins.

2 Place all the sponge ingredients in a food processor and whizz until smooth or beat together in a large bowl.

3 Divide the mixture between the prepared tins and place in a preheated oven, 180°C (350°F), Gas Mark 4, for 12–15 minutes until just firm to the touch and beginning to shrink away from the sides of the tin. Transfer to a wire rack to cool.

4 Beat together all the icing ingredients in a bowl, then spread half over 1 sponge and sandwich together with the remaining sponge. Spread the remaining icing over the top.

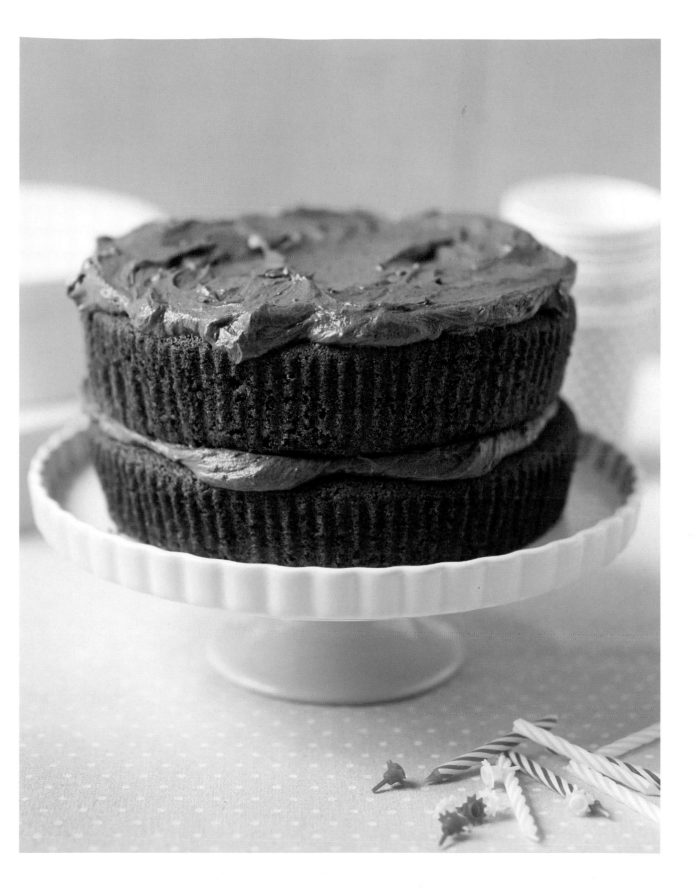

zebra buns

Makes 12

Preparation time 15 minutes, plus cooling

Cooking time 15–18 minutes

250 g (8 oz) butter or margarine, softened

250 g (8 oz) caster sugar

250 g (8 oz) brown rice flour

4 eggs

2 tablespoons cocoa powder

Icing

150 g (5 oz) butter

300 g (10 oz) icing sugar

1 tablespoon cocoa powder

a little milk

1 Line a 12-hole muffin tray with muffin cases.

2 Place the butter or margarine, caster sugar, flour and eggs in a food processor and whizz until pale and smooth or beat together in a large bowl. Spoon out half the mixture into a separate bowl and beat in the cocoa powder.

3 Place the cake mixtures into 2 separate piping bags fitted with plain nozzles. Pipe alternate layers of cake mixture into each case.

4 Place in a preheated oven, 200°C (400°F), Gas Mark 6, for 15–18 minutes until risen and just firm to the touch. Transfer to a wire rack to cool.

5 Beat together all the icing ingredients in a bowl, adding just enough milk to form a soft, smooth consistency. Pipe or spread the icing on to the cooled zebra cakes.

Tips and tricks

You can add orange flavouring to the icing instead of cocoa powder.

chocolate caramel shortbread

Makes 15

Preparation time 20 minutes, plus cooling and chilling

Cooking time 15 minutes

100 g (3½ oz) butter, softened, plus extra for greasing

50 g (2 oz) caster sugar

100 g (3½ oz) brown rice flour

100 g (3½ oz) cornflour

Caramel

100 g (3½ oz) butter

50 g (2 oz) soft light brown sugar

400 g (13 oz) can condensed milk

Topping

100 g (3½ oz) gluten-free white chocolate

100 g (3½ oz) gluten-free plain dark chocolate

1 Grease a 28 x 18 cm (11 x 7 inch) baking tin.

2 Beat together the butter and sugar in a large bowl until pale and fluffy, then stir in the flours until well combined.

3 Press the shortbread into the prepared tin and place in a preheated oven, 200°C (400°F), Gas Mark 6, for 10–12 minutes until golden.

4 Meanwhile, place all the caramel ingredients in a heavy-based saucepan and heat over a low heat until the sugar has dissolved, then cook for 5 minutes, stirring continuously. Remove the pan from the heat and leave to cool slightly.

5 Remove the shortbread base from the oven, then pour the caramel over and leave to cool and set.

6 Melt the white and dark chocolate in separate heatproof bowls set over saucepans of gently simmering water, ensuring the bottoms of the bowls do not touch the water. When the caramel is firm, spoon alternate spoonfuls of the white and dark chocolate over the caramel, tap the tin on the work surface so that the different chocolates join, then use a knife to make swirls in the chocolate.

7 Chill until set, then cut the shortbread into 15 squares.

lemon meringue frozen yogurt

Serves 6

Preparation time 5 minutes, plus freezing

500 g (1 lb) Greek yogurt

2 tablespoons icing sugar

4 tablespoons gluten-free lemon curd

2 meringue nests, crushed

grated rind of 1 lemon

1 Place all the ingredients in a bowl and gently mix together until combined.

2 Transfer the mixture to a freezerproof container and freeze until solid.

super simple vanilla ice cream

Serves 6

Preparation time 5 minutes, plus freezing

400 g (13 oz) can ready-made custard

300 ml (10 fl oz) double cream

This is a very simple recipe that can be adapted by adding fruit purées or flavourings of your choice.

1 Place the custard and cream in a bowl and stir together, then tip the mixture into a freezerproof container.

2 Freeze for 2 hours, then whisk the mixture to remove any ice crystals and return to the freezer for a further 2 hours. Whisk again, then freeze until solid.

lovely lollies

Makes 4

Preparation time 5 minutes, plus freezing

250 g (8 oz) raspberries, defrosted if frozen

2 ripe bananas, chopped

200 g (7 oz) Greek yogurt

3 tablespoons clear honey

1 Place all the ingredients in a food processor or blender and whizz until smooth, then spoon the mixture into 4 lolly moulds.

2 Freeze until solid.

Tips and tricks

These work with any fruit so experiment with different combinations to find your kids' favourite flavour. It's a great way to add fruit to their diet.

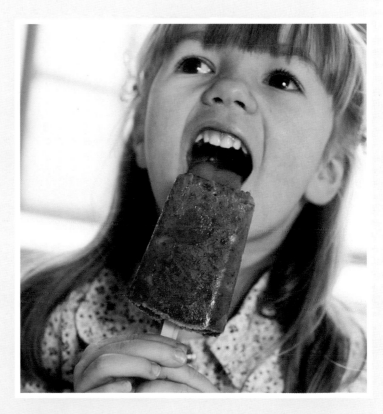

salted caramel popcorn

Serves 4

Preparation time 5 minutes

Cooking time 10 minutes

1 teaspoon sunflower oil

50 g (2 oz) popping corn

200 g (7 oz) caster sugar

25 g (1 oz) knob of butter

sea salt flakes

1 Heat the oil in a large lidded saucepan. Add the popping corn, cover and heat, shaking the pan frequently until the corn has all popped. Tip on to a large sheet of nonstick baking paper.

2 Place the sugar in a large frying pan and heat over a low heat until the sugar has dissolved. Bubble until golden, then stir in the butter. Drizzle the caramel over the popcorn and sprinkle with a little salt.

griddled fruit kebabs

Makes 8

Preparation time 10 minutes, plus soaking

Cooking time 5–6 minutes

40 g (1½ oz) butter, melted

2 tablespoons maple syrup

pinch of ground ginger

2 large firm bananas, cut into chunks

1 papaya, peeled, deseeded and cut into chunks

1 small pineapple, peeled, cored and cut into chunks

cream or yogurt, to serve

1 Pre-soak 8 wooden skewers in water for 30 minutes.

2 Mix together the butter, syrup and ginger in a small bowl. Thread the fruit alternately on to the skewers, then brush with the syrup mixture.

3 Cook under a preheated hot grill or on a barbecue for 5–6 minutes, turning and brushing with syrup occasionally, until golden and beginning to char. Serve with cream or yogurt.

berry smoothie jellies

Serves 4

Preparation time 10 minutes, plus soaking and chilling

Cooking time 3 minutes

6 sheets of leaf gelatine

450 ml (¾ pint) berry smoothie juice

150 ml (¼ pint) fruit yogurt

200 g (7 oz) berries, such as blueberries, raspberries or strawberries

You can use any flavour smoothie to make the jellies – try pairing the smoothies with different fruits. Bear in mind, though, that acidic foods will not give a good jelly set.

1 Soak the gelatine in a bowl of cold water, according to packet instructions, until soft and floppy, then transfer the mixture to a small saucepan and heat very gently until melted. Gradually stir in the smoothie and yogurt.

2 Divide the berries among 4 tall glasses, then pour over the smoothie mixture. Chill until set.

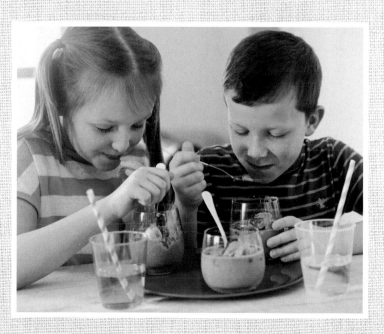

index

acknowledgements

Publisher's credits

Octopus Publishing Group would like to thank all the children featured in this book:
Evie Coughlan, Charlie Killick, Isaac Odeniyi, Sofia Rajah, Ameliah Rajah, Freddie Shaw,
Grace Shaw and Oscar Byrnes Taylor.

Picture credits

Special photography by William Shaw.
Other photography:
Fotolia Tombaky 4 background (used throughout).
Octopus Publishing Group Vanessa Davies 91, 95; Emma Neish 99, 103, 107, 109, 131;
Lis Parsons 71; Craig Robertson 18, 69, 82, 115; William Shaw 14, 15, 27, 39, 44, 60, 68, 75,
83, 84, 114, 119.

Commissioning Editor: **Sarah Ford**
Editor: **Pauline Bache**
Art Director: **Tracy Killick at Tracy Killick Art Direction and Design**
Photographer: **William Shaw**
Home economist: **Louise Blair**
Prop Stylist: **Tony Hutchinson at Refresh**
Picture Library Manager: **Jennifer Veall**
Assistant Production Manager: **John Casey**